CAREFREE CARIBBEAN WEIGHTLOSS

Have fun losing weight with real life, real food, real science, and real people.

Randy Smythe

CAREFREE CARIBBEAN WEIGHTLOSS
Have fun losing weight with real life, real food,
real science and real people.

Library of Congress Cataloging-in-Publication Data
Smythe, Randy.
Carefree Caribbean Weightloss: Have fun losing weight with real life,
real food, real science, and real people.
p. cm.
Includes bibliographical references and index.
ISBN: 978-0-9779098-8-9
    1.   Nutrition   2. Dieting   3. Food preferences.

Everglades Publishers

Disclaimer:
The author of this material has done his best to present accurate and timely information, but cannot guarantee that the information will suit your particular situation. This book is sold with the understanding that the publisher and author are not offering medical advice. The information described herein is for educational purposes only, and may be too difficult for some people. The reader(s) should consult a competent professional if expert assistance is required.

CONTENTS

for Maribel, Damon and Rochelle

Words can't express my gratitude.

One

IN THE BEGINNING...

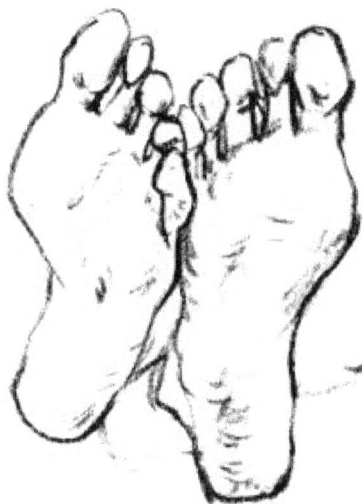

"The problem is not the problem; the problem is your attitude about the problem."
~ Captain Jack Sparrow

"I did it!" She told me that she had proved everyone wrong by losing 10 pounds in one week. She was proud and convinced that she had solved the problem of getting rid of flab in a hurry. How was I supposed to reply? Everything I know about losing weight points to impossible odds of keeping the weight off if it is rapidly lost. "Nice." That was all I could say.

The problem is that she completely misunderstood, or had been completely misled as to how this all works. Weightloss isn't about simply losing pounds, it's about gaining a better life. And in the world of weightloss, life doesn't mean a few days, weeks, or months, it means year after year. For you to lose weight and stay that way for years, there has to be something compelling to keep you on track. Scientific dieting, mathematical formulas, and discipline won't last very long. Here is where the Caribbean Sea works its magic. The culture, the attitude, the music, the way of life of the Caribbean Islands will lead you to a better life, and you don't need to live there. It's not pretending to be someplace else, it's absorbing the very best from your neighbors to the south.

That's what this book is about. Turning to the Caribbean Sea, its culture, its foods, its stress free way of living – this will gradually make you thin. But it will rapidly make you happy. Because this exotic region of the planet is an attitude as much as it is sand and water; you can take it with you wherever you live.

It's no fun being fat, whatever you decide being fat is. Even if you're far from obese, there's a constant feeling of being a disappointment to yourself. When you look around and see streets and offices and airports crowded with critically fat people, it's still no consolation that you're not that fat. There's just no positive feeling to be found. Being overweight is a daily negative experience, often lasting decades.

To make things a lot worse we have a society overwhelmed with dieting mania. You're flooded with information, misinformation, misleading information, infomercials, and outright lies. Literally hundreds of videos are available to watch about people who lost enormous amounts of fat. We have foods that are supposed to help us lose weight. We have health clubs that are supposed to make us thin. We have doctors and therapists to make us thin. We have national campaigns to make us thin. We have slogans and mantras to make us thin. In that none of it works more than a few months, it becomes personal and it becomes emotional.

A couple in their 30's walked up one day and each had on a cast around their waist. Neither of them was obese, but certainly well fed. I asked if they had been in a car accident. Both chuckled at me, for I foolishly didn't know that getting a body cast was the new wave in fat loss. Then there was a successful woman in real estate who complained that for nearly a year she ran and biked each morning, but she couldn't get the remaining 25 pounds off no matter how much dieting or running. Then there was a middle age guy I hadn't seen in many months who showed up one day 50 pounds lighter under the direction of his doctor. It was a year or so later when I saw him again. He had gained at least 100 pounds.

The misery of it all is overwhelming. There are over 200 million people in the US who suffer from being chronically overweight or obese, and no doubt all of them have a sad story to tell. Wouldn't it be great if they could lose that weight, keep it off, and be happy about the process?

This is why the Carefree Caribbean Weightloss system was crafted. It's for the rest of us, including my own 15 year battle with gaining weight. We can't afford to quit work and move to a resort estate in Barbados. We don't have and don't want to have a personal trainer of the stars. Normal people aren't 25 year old thin blondes looking to become even more perfect. In fact, this book is clearly pointed to those who are just regular people who simply want to lose weight.

After many years training elite athletes, I found that there is a way out for all of us. It is from these athletes that the Carefree Weightloss system evolved. With unique training, the use fresh food, and lots of conscious effort at having fun you can manipulate your hormones to work with you, not against you. By blending the Caribbean lifestyle with the authentic flavors of Caribbean meals, a sensible weightloss program for adults evolved. It's a system that has worked wonderfully for centuries.

The people who come to me for help with losing weight find this Carefree system such a relief. It's so simple. There's nothing particularly new about the nutrition side of it other than getting rid of half a century of way too much sugar and starches, industrial toxins, and crazy ideas. There's nothing new about the exercise side of it other than spending more time doing what all of us used to do on the elementary school playground. And the psychological side of it, so important to having any chance of success, is essentially turning to the traditions of Caribbean Island life.

For those of us well north of the Caribbean, the change to an active life and a diet of fresh foods should be no problem other than a big change in attitude. It's different; seemingly too simple to believe that the solution is right before our eyes, right in our neighborhood grocery store.

Just a century ago, every neighborhood in the country was a place where women chatted with friends and exchanged recipes. Food was prepared by mom, served by mom, and mom nurtured the family. Everyday foods were wholesome, meals were the bonding times of the family, and there was no obesity epidemic.

Then fifty years ago western society experienced the onslaught of farming chemicals, artificial sugar, then food additives, then genetically modified crops, then hormones, antibiotics, and more. Today the dream of pre-chemical invasions is like a far off misty horizon. Today we have a devastating obesity and excess weight crisis. Clearly we need to find a solution rooted in the past. That magical time still exists today with the traditional Caribbean life of fresh foods cooked with centuries of refinement on flavor, plus living an active life.

The Carefree Caribbean Weightloss system works because it has served humanity for thousands of years. It's validated by modern science; you'll see dozens of eminent researchers agree. But for you personally, it's is all about taking your time, but really having fun with the process.

Here is a way to fight back and regain a foothold on happiness with a more thin you. Take your time and rebuild yourself on the inside, then let the outside show the results. It's really quite easy, but to do this you have to just let go.

Enjoy the ride.

Two

IT'S IN THE BLOOD

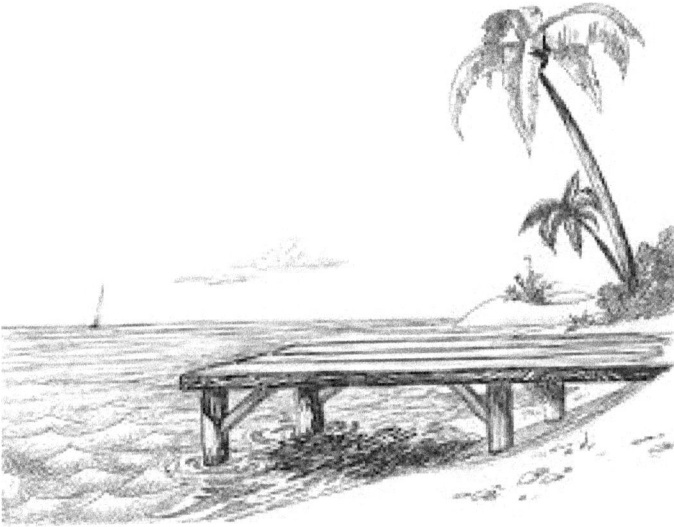

"Oh the places you'll go."
~ Dr. Seuss

The Caribbean Islands are a lot more than palm trees with a warm sea breeze, white sandy beaches, and great music. These tropical lands of the Caribbean Sea have a long tradition of laid-back life; they express an attitude in which Islanders seem to eat and drink whatever they want and miraculously stay thin. As you gaze around while wandering along the coastal streets, it's uncanny how so many people can live and work there and so few are fat. That is, except for the tourists.

What is it? Caribbean Islanders appear to be a very physical people, forever walking, carrying things everywhere, pushing, pulling and lifting. They just seem to be on the go without being in a rush. They seem to eat big meals, drink a lot, even smoke big cigars. You regularly see little yard parties with people laughing and kids playing, where young and old people dance with style. Music blares as you walk down the street. As a complete stranger, more than once you'll be invited in to celebrate. Celebrate what? You'll probably never figure that out, but celebration is an everyday event throughout the region.

For a typical gringo like me, it's overwhelming, especially the attitude of the place. I've been there so many times, met so many great people, experienced life changing romance, tasted life changing foods, sipped the best rum in the world, and learned to dance (badly, to be honest) to fabulous Latin music.

This Caribbean experience opened my eyes to an entirely different way of seeing things. Growing up in Los Angeles with lots of Mexican food and culture, taking vacations just south of the border, I thought that was all there was to Latin life. But after spending time on many of the islands, on Central American beaches, drifting through coastal Colombia and Venezuela… the light bulb turned on. The food, the style of living, the nightlife, the music, the honking horns. Above all, the attitude of the place is most enduring. It's stunning how Islanders live it to the limit.

There is no rule, no uniformity, no measured norm to the Caribbean coastal way of life. Right in the middle of something important happening the electricity shuts off until it decides to come back on again. But everything muddles along in the darkness, life goes on. There is a spirit and vitality none can deny, and it isn't powered by electric wires. It does, however, have a sneaky way of changing everyone who spends time there.

This change of life has convinced me that the dozens of US popular diets we all see will never work to match the shape of Caribbean people. I continue to travel to the islands to work with young baseball stars, and I continue to see a culture and lifestyle that results in predominantly thin people who eat very well and have a lot of fun at everyday life.

It's clear to me that adopting the carefree attitude, much of the traditional Caribbean lifestyle, and a lot of their diet will help you lose weight and enjoy yourself. I have seen it happen to dozens of people. You don't have to adopt it all, you don't have to be there, and you don't have to be a phony. But you do have to change your attitude. Be more active, eat big meals, but it'll be less meat or fish with a lot of vegetables with beans or roots. Over time you'll actually eat less volume of food but the amount of fats you'll eat will increase. This is a culture that features avocados, olive oil, coconut oil, eggs, fatty fish, and plenty of other quality fats.

This isn't miracle food. It is simply fresh food that is higher in fiber, lower in toxins, and all prepared with a flavor to die for. Coupled with a very active lifestyle and moderate exercise, you'll shape yourself a tiny bit each day and lose a pound most weeks. Little by little you'll have a major change in life and a slimmer body to enjoy it with. But more than anything else, it will be fun. There is no calculating calories, no hunger, no white-knuckle discipline, but lots of laid-back laughter.

If the goal of this book was to help you lose weight but to end up stressed and narcissistic, it would never have been written. I wouldn't have had the spark (*chispa* in Spanish) to do all the work it takes to write a book. Instead, this is a guide to show how to lose weight as you live better, eat great food, laugh more, dance more, and hopefully add more romance to your life.

Please, no more diets

This Carefree Caribbean system casts a wide fishing net so as to reap just the right return. It takes in many scientific fundamentals of successful weightloss and avoids many things likely to lead to failure. Even though it is backed by peer reviewed nutrition research, this system is inextricably bound to a place on the planet and its people, their traditions, and the soul (*alma*) of region. Therefore, this isn't a diet. It isn't a bunch of exercises nor is it a psychiatrist's couch. Instead, this is a romantic journey of self-discovery that includes fabulous music, dark chocolate, toasts with red wine and is the very definition of relaxation.

The traditional Caribbean lifestyle is active. Islanders work hard and play hard, all while having a stress-free attitude and a sound night of sleep. The food is almost all local and fresh, thus the avoidance of toxins. The regular exercise tends to be simple, sometimes like on a school playground, and even chaotic. Regularly having a good time is built into the system for many reasons, including hormonal. These components all work together to help you manipulate your hormones to work for you, not against you.

However, the Carefree Caribbean Weightloss system is firmly backed by current science, even the laid-back attitude is essential to weightloss and is based upon peer reviewed science. Stress, sleep, and happiness are of great importance in losing weight, and current research supports this.

The consensus is: stress makes you fat. But this doesn't mean you have to be scientific about relaxing, you don't need to time your fun or measure it. There is no drug or magic elixir or psychiatric treatment to get it. What you do need is to seek fun for many reasons, in this case for the hormonal response that fun has on weightloss. The by-product is a happier life.

All of this fits the checklist of how to overcome the modern pandemic of obesity. All of this fits the checklist of how you lose weight and enjoy the process. All of this fits the checklist of how to make your life better.

None of this Carefree Caribbean system will work without the primary ingredient – an attitude adjustment. Deep inside of each person who seeks a change in life there must be a no-turning-back decision. That decision is a solemn promise to make real change that lasts for years.

You can't have it both ways. Either you make a fundamental change in your life or you'll continue to struggle with excess weight and the stress that makes you miserable. You can't succeed year after year unless you make this journey fun, exciting, and more of an emotional boost than what you have now. Any weightloss system that is just another measurement of carbohydrates or grams of protein will fail in the long run, and it won't be any fun. This one's fun.

This isn't to say that the Carefree weightloss system is the only system that is centered around pesticide-free produce, healthy oils, and low toxin meat. However, it is the only one that is completely interwoven with an existing modern culture that is based on fun, relaxation, and living happily.

From the Mediterranean Sea to the Caribbean Sea

Over the last decade, the Mediterranean Diet has had good success compared to other popular diets. Featuring whole foods, fresh produce, cheese, fish, virgin olive oil, limited sugar, the Mediterranean Diet is a sound one. Unfortunately, it is a diet, not a change in life.

The Carefree system is similar in many ways, but there are several fundamental differences. The Caribbean weightloss system is interwoven with the geography of the region, the different languages, the traditions, and the turbulent history of the place. Even the music of the Caribbean can and should be used to draw you into a reduced stress lifestyle.

Thus the Caribbean system is far from a diet. Instead, it's an outgrowth of Caribbean topography and Island people. There are literally thousands of islands and coastal cities that are five minutes away from lush tropical forests unbothered by man. It is a place you can fly to in a few hours, people you can meet and get to know, and a mixture of lush resort hotels or little beach houses on remote islands.

All around you there are small harbors that seem to have been bypassed by modern life where you can feel the pulse of the region, barter for fresh seafood and produce. You can sleep on a hammock or sit in the sand for hours sipping coconut juice from the coconut tree that shades you. This is an unpretentious life that can change you forever if you let it.

For all of this magical tropic culture to help you lose weight, you don't even have to be there. You can see it in movies and videos, hear it in the music, smell it in fresh food in your kitchen, and taste it every day forever at home. Most of all, the Carefree weightloss system is an attitude that can help you live better whatever you live.

It starts with attitude, it is maintained by attitude, the results are a directly attributed to attitude, and the attitude is a lot of fun. Nutrition itself isn't where most weight loss systems fall apart, it's the attitude, or more specifically, the absence of the right attitude. Therefore, this weightloss system turns traditional dieting upside down. The Carefree system is built to permanently make changes in your life by changing your attitude first. For you to find long term weightloss, you'll need to tap into your creativity and emotions. Almost every diet in existence is a mathematical formula consisting of calories, measured grams of nutrients, and hours of exercise.

What ever happened to emotions? You can't deny the impact emotions have on your decisions, especially when decisions are being made about the way you live. Therefore, you need to somehow balance this most important decision by blending science together with your emotions.

Having fun, enjoying your life, savoring delicious meals, never having to fight through hunger or the feeling of being deprived – this should be your goal. The magic of it all is how humans get thin as they gradually adapt to the simple pleasures shared by ancestors from long ago. We survived an Ice Age, droughts, plagues, wars…we've earned some fun.

Decide to change to something old

The traditional Caribbean diet, made up of a blend of food from multiple cultures and peoples, shows how lost we are today with the Standard American Diet (SAD). It's painful to see how Caribbean people who turn away from their traditional diet and adopt the SAD suffer from the same obesity crisis as North Americans.

Little by little, the SAD is making its way into the islands with devastating effects on health and weight gain. Here at home, fast food, processed food, toxin laden food, and foolish choices in food becomes the chosen diet of immigrants from all over, including those from the Caribbean. The traditional Caribbean diet, being a blend of food and generations of attitudes, is losing to the American diet of obesity.

In tiny cities that dot the coast of this 2,600 mile region, almost no one counts calories much less count grams of carbohydrates. You won't find a meal plan anywhere but a hospital. The medium chain triglycerides of coconut oil are virtually unknown, but the taste is universally loved.

Traditional Islanders eat fresh produce, strange looking fruit, chicken, pig, goat, seafood, and an endless variety of roots. Islanders tend to make a festive occasion out of any meal, and they show no guilt about drinking lots of beer, wine, or dark Caribbean rum. Perhaps more than any region on the planet, life is lived to the fullest on the 7,000 islands known as the West Indies.

The time has come to make up your mind to let the centuries old Caribbean way of life help you. In your own way, live more like the traditional Islanders, be more active like them, enjoy your relaxation more like them. Treat yourself to traditional Caribbean style of cooking.

The Carefree system will then take away problematic foods such as modern industrial grains, pesticide filled produce, toxin laden seafood, antibiotic laden meat, sugar loaded foods, processed foods, and the nightmare of modern processed fats. You'll find that the traditional diet throughout the entire Caribbean culture avoids these foods as Islanders prefer the simple and local foods made by grandmother.

However, there are some favorites of traditional the Caribbean diet that don't fit with the Carefree weightloss system. The modern world has contaminated seafood, and sadly altered Caribbean seafood into a toxin laden staple. You'll need to substitute Wild Alaskan Salmon, cold water trout, and select shellfish to steer clear of most toxins.

Free range meat and chicken will need to replace your standard fare, and careful shopping will be needed to steer clear of the worst toxin loaded produce. But never fear, this is easily done with the information provided in the Carefree system along with easy links to sourcing the best and safest (see chapter 10). Don't worry, overall the cost will be significantly less than what you spend now when you figure in the savings inherent in the simplicity of Caribbean foods.

Fruit of the angels

When Columbus arrived in the West Indies he found a strange melon-like plant he called "fruit of the angels" which we know to be papaya. Hidden within the mild taste of Caribbean red papaya is a jolt of protein-digesting enzymes that are a great help to weightloss.[1] My wife grew up in coastal Venezuela and never heard of proteolytic papaya enzymes, but she follows family tradition and serves up papaya at the first sign of stomach ache, and she joins millions of Latinas who regularly eat papaya to delay onset of wrinkles.

Pineapple trees flourish throughout the region and research shows that fresh pineapple features the digestive enzyme bromelain that aids in weightloss.[2] Bromelain is a potent anti-inflammatory that stimulates the digestion process, but don't expect the Islanders to know of this. Throughout the Caribbean pineapple is an everyday fare because it tastes great and grandmother cooks with it.

Coconut trees dominate the Central America shoreline today just as when Columbus landed. Not only was coconut "meat" eaten, but the juice was relished, and the oil became the preferred "medicine" for numerous ailments. Today clinical research shows that cancer, heart disease, arthritis, diabetes, and many other western degenerative diseases are almost unheard of among cultures that rely on coconut for a large part of their diet.[3] Coconut oil can aid in weightloss goals despite the fact that it has been measured to have 92% saturated fat.

Conventional wisdom tells us that saturated fats are supposed to cause heart disease. However, the traditional Caribbean diet is rich in saturated fats and there are very low levels of heart disease. By cultural accident it turns out that the traditional Caribbean Island diet is way ahead of scientific research in terms of guidelines for quality fat consumption. As you'll see, ample coconut and other quality fats are a key to weightloss and health, plus the taste of coconut oil is fabulous. Coconut oil is excellent for cooking flavorful tropical dishes, in part because it can be heated much higher than olive oil without losing nutrient value.

At sundown in these sun-drenched islands, the creamy juice of coconut is strained, then blended with fresh juice from pineapple. Crushed ice is added along with a shot of Caribbean rum. The result is the glory of the *Pina Colada*, absolute proof that life is good.

Systematic failure

The stress of modern life makes us fat. In her book on the subject, Dr. Pamela Peeke states, "Even if you usually eat well and exercise, chronic high stress can prevent you from losing weight, or even add pounds."[4] We add stress by eating meals standing up or even as we drive. We build up stress because we sleep less, and that sleep is significantly interrupted by ambient light from phones, clocks, and meters. We drink vast amounts of caffeinated coffee well into the night, sip soft drinks, energy drinks, and cups of hidden sweeteners to add to everyday stress.

After all of this self-induced stress we wonder why adrenal fatigue is rampant and why weightloss gets stalled despite strict dieting and hours of exercise. Studies clearly show that the things we eat and drink lead to adrenal fatigue, and this leads to weight gain.[5] Now the problem becomes critical as we become stressed about having so much stress.

Excessive stress triggers the hormonal release of cortisol which "protects us from famine" by storing abdominal fat. The presence of cortisol then suppresses leptin hormone levels, raises ghrelin hormone levels that reduce fat metabolism and raise hunger. Stress further triggers more hormonal chaos as insulin levels remain high, like a car alarm continually blaring even though there is no danger. The insulin levels remain high, the body stays on emergency alert, abdominal fat is stored, and the result is that you feel hungry and miserable as you gain more weight.

Another contributing factor to failure in weightloss is the utter punishment of it all. You tell yourself that you made yourself fat. You feel you've been eating like a pig, too lazy to exercise, and now you can't eat the foods you crave. You feel you have to starve yourself using white-knuckle discipline to get by on a ridiculously low amount of calories. Like a zombie you stare at the clock counting the minutes until you can eat your prescribed bird food snack. Is there any wonder why diets fail?

In our world that creates stress, the SAD then triggers fat storage. It's the wrong industrial carbohydrates, the wrong chemically treated industrial meats, the wrong synthetic chemical laden produce, the wrong processed seed oil, the wrong antibiotic laden dairy products, the wrong micro-biome destructive industrial chemicals we consume, all featured in the SAD. This is the recipe for getting fat, staying fat and miserable.[6] In order to overcome the SAD nightmare, you are told to count calories. They are important, but not *the* important measurement for weightloss. This is because we've all been fooled into thinking that all calories are created equal. Not true! Clean fresh food that's brimming with nutrients provides much more energy and sensation than industrially processed calories so lacking in nutrients. Your body reacts differently to different calories; differently when crunching, tasting, and smelling a fresh apple than taking a spoonful of powdered apple concentrate.

The calorie counting narrative is that 500 calories of salmon sautéed in olive oil on top of a fresh garden salad is somehow the same as a 500 calorie sandwich of processed turkey-ham on industrial bread lathered with preservative laden mayonnaise. Now is the time to stop this madness and let quality, not calorie counting rule the day. Shift your focus to quality of food and quality of life.

No one bothered to mention to you that the foods you have been eating most of your life, even "health" foods are programmed to make you fat. Conventional wisdom screams that all belly fat is caused by gluttony; excess calories make you fat. No one tells you about the recent discovery of obesogens in pesticide laden food and everyday environmental chemicals. Simply put, various chemistry lab compounds that find their way into your food and environment to make you fat.[7] Therefore, standard grocery store spinach and kale, repeatedly sprayed with pesticides can have a toxic load triggering fat storage many times worse than a bowl of homemade ice cream.

Modern life of consuming commercial foods that are swimming in man-made chemicals; this must change if you are to change your life and become happy with yourself. It's clear that these synthetic chemical compounds are the primary reason that the Centers for Disease Control states that three out of four Americans are either overweight or obese.

In fact, it's worse. The clinical definition of overweight has moved up so that a borderline overweight person today would have been labeled critically overweight by standards half a century ago.

Is there any way out of this? A resounding yes!

Caribbean life in Chicago

"Wine is constant proof that God loves us and loves to see us happy."
   ~ Benjamin Franklin

Live and enjoy the Caribbean life, even if its winter and you live in Chicago. It's an attitude. It's a mindset, it's a metaphor, and it's a method to overcome the madness that surrounds you. It will make you feel better, eat better, exercise better, and look better. Go ahead, turn on some music and sip a glass of sangria as you cook.

Red wine's abundance of resveratrol has been clinically found to help metabolize fat, plus it makes the evening a whole lot more fun.[8] Taken in moderation, you'll come out slim, singing different songs, and actually eating larger meals, although most of it will be great tasting vegetables.

In your own neighborhood, live as a Caribbean Islander would. You'll soon discover the amazing results from enjoying the Caribbean tradition of eating roots and those iconic green bananas (plantains). These resistant starches, so popular in Hispanic culture, are a unique type of high fiber carbohydrate that are difficult for digestive enzymes to break down. Resistant starches travel along the small intestine straight to the colon without being absorbed as glucose. They resist typical intestinal breakdown and instead are metabolized by gut flora in the colon. A moderate amount of these filling starches provide energy without the excess being turned into body fat.

The russet potato, first cooked then cooled, is also a resistant starch, but it comes from the worst of our mass chemical saturation of farmland. The USDA Pesticide Data Program lists 35 different pesticides in conventional potatoes, 12 of which are hormone disruptors. The primary herbicide used on russet (white potatoes) is lethal chlorpropham, but because russets grow underground, they soak in many other pesticides along with petroleum based fertilizers. Clearly this would be a bad choice when traditional Caribbean roots such as yuca along with plantains form the majority of Islander dietary starches. These resistant starches have none of the industrial contaminants so common in russet potatoes.

The tremendous flavor of island herbs and spices will ruin you – you'll never be able to go back to bland foods again. You'll also be ruined by the base of many Caribbean dishes, called *sofrito*. It is a sauté of garlic, onion, bell pepper and whatever else might be on hand, plus a blend of herbs. Within a few minutes the blend of herbs cooked into the *sofrito* creates a taste and aroma that transends the plate of vegetables and fish or meat. It is a life changing sauce. People who hate vegetables line up for more when prepared the *sofrito* way.

With *sofrito* (or the Colombian equivalent *hogao*) in your life the amount of vegetables you'll eat will triple or quadruple. No one will tell you to and no one will measure anything, but the Caribbean flavors of the meat, fish, roots, and vegetables will blend with the *sofrito*, and then overwhelm you.

Like your ancestors you'll have a physical connection with what you eat, not just something bland that's heaped on your plate. When you buy the produce, chop it, cook it, serve it, then savor it, you'll undoubtedly appreciate it lot more than eating something out of a Styrofoam container. The Caribbean attitude adjustment takes place in the care as well as extra moments of your own cooking creativity it will take. But this is what the traditional Caribbean meal consists of, and it is all part of enjoying a new way of living and eating.

Who came up with the idea of tasteless steamed vegetables? Go Caribbean. There is an incredible blend of flavors and textures when vegetables are prepared the Caribbean way. These vegetables, herbs, roots, and spices are easy to find at your grocery store. Eggplant, cabbage, squash, pumpkin, cucumber, green beans, okra, beets, and other staples are prepared in ways that are layered with flavor, the opposite of North American culinary styles. They are quick and easy to chop up and make into your own personalized *sofrito*. You can prepare these Caribbean dishes in your apartment in New York or rural Missouri. If you have very basic pots and pans and very basic cooking experience you can make Caribbean food tonight.

Prepare to learn all about herbs and spices. Although Trinidad, Jamaica, and Mexico love super-hot pepper foods, most Islanders shun the super-hot and go for layers of flavor instead. Either way, science now shows us that the liberal use of cinnamon, turmeric, cumin, cayenne pepper and other everyday Caribbean spices play an important role in weightloss, in a large part due to raising the metabolism.[9] The result is food that smells amazing, features a bright bouquet of colors, tastes out of this world, and helps to get you thin.

Caribbean meals have somehow evolved to be heaven sent for those wishing to lose weight and body fat. The variety is never ending; from English tradition, to French, to Spanish, to Asian, to African. But each tends to rely on a similar starting point with cultural taste differences.

A Caribbean plate is roughly divided into three parts: a protein, a starch, and a vegetable. Often the parts are combined as in a hearty soup, a stir fly, or a slow cooked stew. Frequently the meat, fish, yuca, corn, and sweet potato (*batata*) are cooked on a barbeque (*plancha*). Applying what you've learned, you'll almost always have a garden salad as well. The tradition of changing flavor and altering texture means that every meal will be uniquely different from the day before.

Carefree life takes a little effort

Caribbean life is the opposite of stressful life but you have to live it. The Carefree system actively teaches you how to live with mind over matter. "I don't mind and it don't matter."

Oddly enough, it takes time and effort to live carefree. You need to start with information, learning about food, shopping, stress reduction, exercise, and having more fun. Next, you'll need to get the ingredients in your kitchen, have the recipes nearby (chapter 9), and have basic pots and pans to use. In this case, basic means an old fashioned cast iron frypan, a cast iron sauté pan, and even a big cast iron pot for cooking soup.

It's highly recommended that you set up a way to listen to Caribbean music as you cook. This musical decision adds an important component to the entire cultural adaptation. This is a new system you'll be adapting to and it's best done by diving in. The music blends with the different foods, the aromas, and the attitude it takes to be laid back.

It always helps to look over YouTube to see what the endless variety of Caribbean cooking looks like and the reaction of those feasting of the meals. This Carefree system depends on you firing up your creativity, and YouTube is an excellent way to start. YouTube will also show you how to dance with abandon to great Latin music, even if you dance alone. Like a little kid, you have to let yourself fall into the story with reckless abandon.

There will be frustration along the way as you navigate contradictory information. For example, even though you'll find that beets are a tremendous benefit to weightloss, you have to eliminate jars of pickled beets with their preservatives and sugars. Even when you find a source of fresh beets, you'll need to read in advance to know most grocery store beets are loaded with chemical pesticides. After a while you'll know that the vast majority of the food you buy is fine from the local grocery store, even though meat, beets and several others will need to be organic. Fortunately, more and more grocery stores offer an organic section to make it easier for careful shoppers.

Most people find it awkward or just strange getting adjusted to the practice of nutritional timing. This is about "shocking" the body with intermittent fasting. It involves paying attention to the amount of time you need to go without eating anything between meals. There will even be times where you purposely miss a meal or two. In this way you can trick hormones into firing when you want them to in order to better serve your weightloss plan.

It would be easy to panic hearing of this and make a lot out of nothing. Eating nothing for four hours after a meal and especially nothing after an early dinner really isn't difficult. There's nothing to fear. With the right foods and the right anti-hunger green tea, these few hour fasts are a breeze resulting in virtually zero hunger.

Intermittent fasting really works when you stick to it. It is actually a series of mini-fasts that stimulate the metabolization of body fat.[10] You'll trigger a hormonal reaction that sends a jolt of human growth hormone (HGH) to build lean muscle tissue, and the very creation of HGH metabolizes fat. You don't need to go a full day without food and you never need to starve yourself. In reality, it is based upon the way Islanders have lived for centuries, working hard for hours then eating a big full meal.

Take time to adjust to green tea, a critical component to the Carefree system. You can actually feel it take away hunger right after you drink it. It is imported from Asia and it has a 4,500 year tradition of serving humanity. Obviously Chinese green tea isn't part of the Caribbean tradition but fits nicely into the weightloss program.

Green tea's phytonutrients will go to work triggering several hormones, including the gut hormone CCK, a messenger to the brain reporting that you have adequate food in your system. International studies confirm that green tea has many hormonal balancing benefits.[11] Even though it boosts energy somewhat similar to caffeine, it has only about 5% of the caffeine as coffee when consumed as iced tea. It has a great exotic flavor, brings a light surge of energy, keeps you hydrated, and tricks you into having a little bit of highly beneficial lemon or lime several times per day.

Where else are you going to find a weightloss treatment that removes hunger pangs, has centuries of service to health, and tastes great with ice?

Make your line in the Caribbean sand

It isn't chanting ancient Buddhist mantras, just a series of long calm walks. Before you change one bite in your current eating habits, before you sweat one droplet, you owe it to yourself to walk alone, no particular destination. Walk far and think deeply. No music, no distractions, nothing to interrupt your thinking.

Figure out what is really making you unhappy. What would you need to do to make things better right away, then what would be needed to make it better for years? What would you be willing to give up, and what would you permanently change in your life? What would be the easiest thing to do, and what would be the easiest thing to stop doing?

Here is the way to truly make your line in the sand, an intelligent life decision where you say, "I've made up my mind and I won't go back." This should stir your soul, almost like a change in religion.

Your decision on who you are and how you wish to live your life is your own compass. If part of that decision is that you don't want to live fat any more, you're in the right place. Your decision to change is well backed up by science, has centuries of successful implementation, and with several million people who practice this healthful lifestyle every day.

No more yo-yo diets, no more buying magic liquids or powders that never work but eventually make you feel worse. No more losing weight rapidly followed by a long term weight gain. Stop doing this to yourself! Refuse to let the same thing happen over and over again. Stop bashing your self-esteem ever more as you flounder.

Make up your mind to dump the guilt, get rid of regrets, forgive the transgressions. Whatever happened in the past is now ancient history to you. It was part of what made you. If you are overweight, even a lot overweight, this wasn't genetically determined like having blue eyes. Your current shape doesn't determine who you will be or how you will live in the future. Find strength from whatever has happened in the past and begin today to change yourself into something better.

One thing that will give you strength will be your stern refusal to follow a foolish diet. There is a psychological self-flagellation about dieting as it exists today. Counting calories and starving yourself, trying to fit into other people's mold made for you…this will forever cause you pain and humiliation. Starving yourself with discipline, drugs or surgery won't change your thinking process – this requires an attitude adjustment. The goal should be to eat great flavorful food in moderation, enjoy it to the hilt, never feel deprived, never feel hungry, never feel weak, and never feel ashamed of yourself. For all of this, you might as well give this Caribbean system a thorough try.

It's time to enjoy life

I got my toes in the water, ass in the sand
Not a worry in the world, a cold beer in my hand
Life is good today. Life is good today.
     ~ Zac Brown Band

Pretend for a moment that you have made your life changing decision. All the obstacles along the way have been brushed away by the Tooth Fairy who has set you free. No longer tied to the mast, you're free of all worldly responsibilities. If you think long and hard in this manner it's a lot of fun. Go ahead, you have the right to dream as much as you want.

Pretend that you are sipping your *Pina Colada* as you dig your toes in the sand, waiting for the waitress to bring the meal you ordered as you sit without a care in the world. Enjoy the change in attitude, especially the way you pardoned yourself for all past crimes and omissions. The only thing you are disciplined about now is relaxing, having fun, and enjoying the life you've missed. You can enjoy a laid-back Caribbean attitude back home. You can enjoy the food, the music, the rum and you don't have to leave your home to do so. Take your shoes off now and wiggle your toes.

It is easy if you will just let yourself go. Enjoy your emotional make-over and your island food for three months to adapt yourself, little by little, to this style of life. The first month is easy. After three months it will be easy to do it again for the next three months, and the whole year, and several years. Everything will fall into place as long as you have the right attitude.

Start by making a concentrated effort to celebrate, to enjoy, to listen to the music. Really, truly try to find ways to plug fun into your life. Make sure that many times every day you do something different that you really like but talked yourself out of in the past. Come on, smile more. Sing real loudly in the shower. Repeat, "I don't mind and it don't matter."

Don't fear the change in cooking. Caribbean food preparation is simple, pretty much the opposite of Julia Child or Gordon Ramsay. Try to have most of the needed ingredients but if not, so what. Measure by eyeball and mostly by hand. Chop onion, garlic, and produce, cook in a little coconut oil or olive oil. Toss in meat, add flavorful seasoning, sauté until you're satisfied, taste and serve. Have some berries and dark chocolate for desert, all the while sipping inexpensive red wine (so plentiful in resveratrol.) With music blaring as no one is looking, dance to *bachata* music on your YouTube favorites. It's that easy.

This is not going to cost more, in fact it'll reduce overall food expenditure significantly. The "cost" isn't money, but time. Before you panic and claim that you're already too busy, stop. Think this through. If you are thoroughly frustrated with your shape and your soul-killing life, here is a golden opportunity to get out of the trap and have lots of fun in the process. The time is mostly cutting vegetables and washing up the kitchen after the meal. You can greatly reduce the time it takes by cutting a mass of vegetables then freezing them in small freezer jars to use as needed. A large pot of Caribbean soup can easily be frozen in many meal size jars, ready to serve minutes after you arrive home late from work.

There is no excuse for claiming that it takes too much time when you compare it to the despair of not being able to shed weight seemingly glued to you. You don't need to drive all over town looking for strange ingredients, they are right in front of you. Special items can easily be ordered online. Even the regular exercise, specifically selected because it triggers hormonal balance and is fun to do, can be done in 30 minutes at home, sometimes even as your meal is cooking. The time has come to stop making excuses. The time has come to make a change.

Therefore, change your thinking from diet to living better. Change from fearing starvation into forcing yourself to do something different and interesting. Stop fearing exercise and just go outside and walk for a while. Make up your mind that you can and will succeed for three months, even if you only succeed a little each day.

Three

A CAREFREE BRAIN

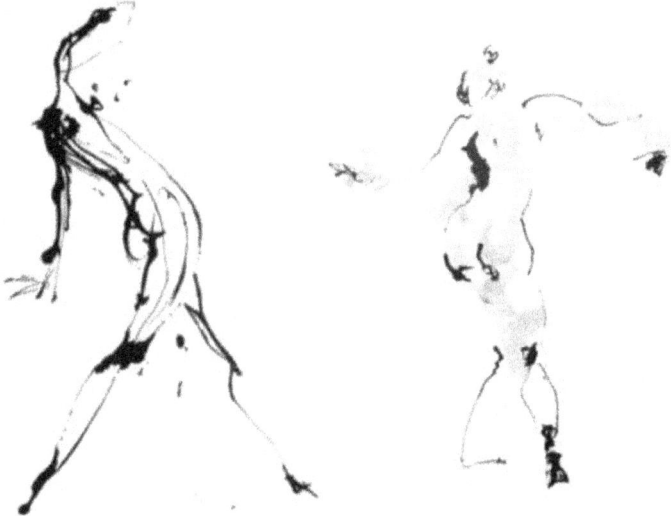

"Twenty years from now you will be more disappointed by the things that you didn't do than by the ones you did do, so throw off the bowlines, sail away from safe harbor, catch the trade winds in your sails. Explore, dream, discover."

~ Mark Twain

There are two popular narratives about your ability to lose weight. One is that you only need to pay for a new diet or new exercise program and your fat will melt away into the ozone. The other is that you're screwed – science has you by the throat and you have no escape.

Consider the terrifying results of this meta-analysis published in 2007. A landmark nine-year study by UCLA researchers found that of over 278,000 obese patients, "maintaining weight loss was rare and the probability of achieving normal weight was extremely low." Researchers led by Professor Traci Mann analyzed 31 clinical diet studies lasting four or more years and concluded the following, "You can initially lose five to

10 percent of your weight on any number of diets, but then the weight comes back." Mann and her research team found that between 89 to 97 percent of critically overweight people in the midst of a diet will fail. The study went on to point out that the chances for an obese woman in any given year to return to normal weight was calculated at 1 in 124. The chances of obese men to return to normal weight was 1 in 210.[1]

Happily, there is a third way of seeing things. Caribbean Islanders have lived more than 3,000 years maintaining a rigorous life with ample native food resulting in a mass of healthy people. North Americans need to find a way to copy this simple but active way of life that flourishes just 100 miles from our southern shores. Sadly, instead of reaching out to learn all we can about Caribbean culture and diet, we make matters worse by looking to the latest Hollywood fad. Then our blindness is compounded as we allow ourselves to be swallowed up by stress.

Weight gain, the inability of dieting to lose weight and keep it off, and the ineffectiveness of exercise programs to rid us of excess weight – all of this makes for a depressing view of life. At the same time, the stresses of everyday life grinds us all down. Pressure from work, pressure from family, pressure to live up to self-imposed expectations, pressure to complete long overdue tasks, pressure to be on time through unrelenting traffic.

The stresses inevitably take on a life of their own, regardless of origin. The stress itself destroys sought after success that is supposedly made up of health and a sense of meaning in life. Like some Greek tragedy, the stress that works to dominate us does so with our helpful hands. All of this stress feeds yet more stress in a falling domino action that triggers hormones to store visceral fat.

Misunderstanding

As you look in the mirror you might hate what you see. You might fear standing on the weight scale for yet another setback. There you are, late in the day, drained of energy as you support the weight of the world on your shoulders and hips. You sip coffee, nibble at processed snacks, feel the burn of stomach discomfort, eat again and get more discomfort, and then push yourself through the day. You sleep badly, yet again, then wake the next morning to repeat it all day after day. Why? The answer is the way you've misunderstood how to be happy and healthy. Get away from all the depressing viewpoints and look for a realistic solution.

Dream of living a new Caribbean life of freedom, then live it right where you are. Maybe someday you can get on a plane and fly there for an extended life away from the madness. But in the meantime, follow the slogan, "act as if until you become." Practice feeling free, practice being happy. Weightloss at the personal level is not a scientific discussion or formula; it's a feeling that becomes an attitude. Then everything after that falls into place.

In order to develop the attitude that will carry you through four years of weightloss and maintenance of a better, thinner you, start by refusing. Refuse to be tricked by slick marketing, old wives' tales, conventional wisdom, and stupid claims such as, "they say that..."

Before you can start to fix yourself, you have to stop beating yourself up with foolish notions and destructive habits. In this case, the needed action is for you to refuse to accept the misinformation that surrounds you. Based on the landmark UCLA study on ineffective dieting, who in their right mind would trust their health and wellbeing to a program where nine out of ten people fail? That would be the opposite of playing the odds to succeed.

To be fair, there are diets that succeed in a laboratory or hospital setting, and these diets run the gamut of low fat, low carb, high protein, prescribed exercise with diet, and lots of diets in between. Hooray! 20, 30, 40, or even 50 pounds vanish within a couple of months. But then the patient gets unhooked and released from the hospital. All hell breaks loose as they step back into the real world after living in a bubble.

What went wrong? Did the patient fail or did the diet fail? Essentially, the diet authors failed to understand two modern realities:

First, they misunderstood tectonic shift in post-industrial society where men, women and children spend long hours each day at work, at school, at day care, and in their car. The problem is time. Eating has shifted from home cooked meals to industrial food: the foods we consume are predominantly pre-packaged and industrially prepared. They are eaten quickly at home, or eaten in a car, or eaten in a fast food restaurant.

Second, they misunderstood the enormous power of marketing. Modern society is so saturated with instant gratification that the UCLA model of a four year threshold of a diet to succeed is never actually considered. Sure, a diet can work for a few weeks, and no doubt some of them work for several months. However, in a competitive market society, why bother encouraging people to take off half a pound each week (which comes out to 26 pounds per year) when the competition is selling their diet as getting rid of 26 pounds in a month.

The only sane way for you to make it through this minefield of misinformation is to absolutely refuse to do the same things as other people. Accept reality; diets don't work. Be unique and find a different way to gradually lose weight for four years. This will defy the odds and will change your life.

Caloric obsession

The amount of calories consumed has much less to do with the epidemic of obesity than how the specific foods trigger hormonal reactions. Excessive calories are important; you can't ignore the problem of eating too much. Sumo wrestlers in Japan eat good clean food in enormous quantities and then grow enormously fat. But there is a point of balance, of sanity, of living an active life, a life of moderation that is conducive to weightloss.

Take control of your food quality as much as you can. There is no such thing as perfect or truly organic food unless grown and prepared in a bubble. Once you take control, it's quality that counts, not quantity of calories. If 80% of your food is as good as you can get, you'll be doing much better than your peers. Overall, with good quality ingredients and great Caribbean taste, by far most of your food will be the opposite of the SAD. However, there is the problem of dining out.

Without question, the worst choice we make in food quality comes from dining at restaurants. We are a nation that relies on restaurants of all kinds, and excessive dining at restaurants makes us fat. This is a given to the formula of helping yourself and taking control. Restaurants lull you into thinking you are ordering foods that help you control your weight (low calorie, low sodium, low fat) when you actually make yourself a little fatter every time you dine out. Even when you carefully order healthful restaurant meals – the industrial bread, the pesticide loaded salad and vegetables, the industrial chicken breast, the cooking oils, the sauce and dressing – all contribute to weight gain.

You won't get fat eating at a restaurant and watching what you eat on occasions, but until you are disciplined about restaurants, they will ruin your dreams of weightloss.

Selling obesity

"A lie told often enough becomes the truth."
~ Vladimir Lenin

There are a lot of people who are thrilled with our obesity epidemic. If a magic wand were to wave away this epidemic today, tomorrow there would be an economic disaster. Our fat society requires a huge service industry. This is why the weightloss industry is a key player in the economy funding doctors, nurses, medical office workers, personal trainers, diet powder packagers, insurance salesmen, office landscapers, truck drivers, bookkeepers, advertising executives, lawyers, and funeral parlor workers. The annual tally is $586.3 billion according to *Marketsandmarkets.com*.[2]

This huge industry spends lavishly on advertising. To rival Burger King and Domino's pizza ads, the weightloss industry spends $20 billion each year hiring the same advertising agencies that just finished a marketing campaign for breakfast cereal or Snickers bars. There are so many, many overweight Americans that the weightloss industry has a market of over 220 million people to serve, with 69% of adults over 20 years of age being listed as clinically overweight or obese according to the Centers for Disease Control (CDC).[3]

Over 100 million Americans repeatedly purchase weightloss foods and supplements, with a surprisingly similar amount spent on these in each demographic group from 18 to 65 years of age. They get almost nothing for their money. Numerous studies, concurring with the landmark UCLA meta-analysis, show that within three years over 90% of diet and exercise clients will be flabby once again.

It's so bad that research published in the *International Journal of Obesity* makes a strong argument that dieting makes people get fatter.[4] We've become so habitual about diets that as the diet runs out of gas, we simply accept the resulting weight gain as if it is part of the process. If dozens of various diets won't help you, and thousands of gyms won't get rid of fat and keep it off for more than three years, why do Americans spend $583.3 billion in a failing effort to lose weight?

It all boils down to misinformation. Diet and exercise by themselves, no matter how you blend them, won't produce long range weight loss. If you let yourself into the diet mindset, a multi-billion dollar industry will eat you alive. With a baited hook stuck in your lip, you'll be reeled in to believe that two weeks from today all of your problems with weight will be solved. The word "diet" binds you to the marketing slogans and celebrity endorsements of an industry that gets you and your credit card to act on smoke and mirrors. Soon you'll find that you don't have a physical problem; the real problem is drumming up the courage to absolutely refuse the misinformation they are pushing.

How did we get so far off track?

Look at the list of stupid weightloss solutions we buy into. You can get a surgically installed patch sewn on your tongue to make eating a painful chore; you can opt for liposuction; or you can join 199,999 other people each year and get your stomach stapled in bariatric surgery. You can take

Adderall (that wonderful drug for attention that is functionally identical to crystal meth) to quell your appetite and raise your metabolism until the minor problem of addiction takes over your life.

You can go old-school and try bulimia, where sticking a finger down your throat will get you to vomit up your last meal, triggering hormonal hell along with raw stomach acids to rot your teeth. You can go modern Hollywood and take Ipecac syrup which makes you vomit without using your finger, but you still get the same hormonal and stomach acid disaster. Why not try urine injections that trick the body into burning calories faster? Believe it or not, people even drink their urine in the faint hope of losing weight.

There's always the Beyoncé inspired 11 day Lemonade Diet where you exist on lemon juice and maple syrup and lose 20 pounds. If you're impatient with waiting 11 days, for a substantial fee a specialist will help you lose 10 pounds in three days; all you do is swallow mysterious pills, starve, and basically live in the bathroom. It's as if our brains are flushed down the toilet in the process. Standing with feet hanging off the edge of the bathroom scale, millions peer at the number begging for the reading to dip just a little more. However, virtually every human who loses bathroom weight knows intuitively that the weight scale will bounce back up in a day or so. But we do it anyway.

We blindly accept the quick fix solutions sold to us with a straight face. The advertising campaigns of past efforts to sell another weightloss product litter the brain with worn-out phrases. Instantly, a weight problem that has taken years to develop is miraculously going to vanish in 10 days, painlessly, and you get to eat everything you want, just as long as you buy the magic powder. And we buy it.

Islanders who live a traditional tropical life and work hard each day don't live this way. They have not slipped so far off track, not become delusional, not been lured into yet another yo-yo diet. We have. For years we've been surrounded by absurd notions of weightloss that come into and out of fashion like new shoe styles. These notions and their ridiculous claims have caused much misery and scarred the psyche of a generation.

Once you refuse to be part of the madness, you can fix things with a simple and functional long range plan. The plan that works starts with a no-turning-back attitude adjustment. No more living in a swamp of misinformation and stress. Eat real healthful fresh foods, exercise regularly, thoroughly enjoy life, and the result will be that you live more like the carefree souls of the Caribbean. You'll lose weight a little at a time, and you'll have a lot of fun doing it.

False models

If you could have a perfect body but had to live a stress filled life or live in a way that would make you unhappier than you are today, clearly this would be something to avoid. It's foolish to think in this way. Your search for sane weightloss should be with the picture of you being you, just slimmed down, but with a big smile. This can happen quite easily if you accept simplicity as your guide.

You're probably not anthropomorphically built to physically match what Hollywood tells you the ideal look is. The problem isn't you, it's Hollywood. The chiseled abs, or silicon stuffed breasts, or rippling biceps, all on a body that is tanned and beautiful – this is the photoshopped image you're supposed to live up to. It is a modern health disaster that almost guarantees unhappiness. Ask yourself, are bodybuilders and Hollywood models happy and satisfied with life?

The false models of what we're all supposed to look like cause a real problem. The phony bodies presented by the cameras get us all to believe that this is reality, something that exists in nature. In no time it has you wondering what you can do to look like that. It is my belief that simplicity is what will make you happy and enjoy what you've got, especially if what you've got is getting better little by little. Even though I was born and raised near Hollywood (Culver City), I don't see Hollywood offering one droplet of simplicity. However, simplicity comes by the boatload in the Caribbean; it is the very definition of Caribbean life. You can see it, you can meet the people who live it, you can model your life back home after it. And it is based upon a life of seeking enjoyment, including the enjoyment of losing weight a little at a time.

Refuse to be bothered by the destructive Hollywood inspired concept of what shape you should be. Replace it with a laid-back lifestyle of Islanders who basically live a life that is built upon real food, hard physical work, great friends and having a good time. This is the way to develop a better body and enjoy the process.

For the love of sweat

Three months of the Carefree system will lead to loss of weight, loss of body fat, a raise in your metabolism, a considerable boost in energy, and more enjoyment of simple fun times. But dietary changes need to be interwoven with exercise. It's important to understand how the two fit together, as dieting alone won't work and exercise alone won't work. It is the combination that does the job when you find a way to also reduce stress. The problem comes with the question, "What exercise?"

There are dozens of exercise programs out there for you to choose from. Clearly, your exercise program should be what you want, not what you are told is good for you. The program can vary greatly, but the most important part of it is to enjoy it so you want to continue with it. If you have fun with it, you'll come back for more. If it is so intense and painful that you fear it, you'll stop doing it. If it is what conventional wisdom tells you to do but you hate it, you'll be guaranteed to fail.

The number one goal of exercise is...you need to come back and do it again soon. Almost any kind of workout will help your blood circulation, bone density, energy level, and help improve your sleep. However, it is important that two elements are part of what you do each time you exercise: balance and resistance.

Work on your balance every time even if it is walking with a dictionary balanced on your head, or balancing a broom stick in your hand, or walking sideways on a curb. Add regular bouts of resistance. That can mean a dozen push-ups or stepping on and off a park bench. Millions people love the clanking of weight plates in a gym, the sound and the smell can be addictive for those with a sports background. If yoga is for you, go for it. Millions love the solitude of lacing up running shoes and taking off for a jog. Bike riders are usually bored with everything until they hear the sound of a bike, then they get goosebumps.

The key is to just include something that challenges your balance and something with resistance along with your favorite exercise. Whatever it is, find what you like the most and do it your way to your satisfaction. 30 minutes a few times per week is great, no matter how intense you like it. 30 minutes is a great amount of time because it's hard to say you can't find the time. 30 minutes is great because it's hard to dread it, especially if it has a few interesting balance exercises included.

Refuse to be tricked by health clubs

Our $75 billion health club industry can be great if that is the magnet that draws you into consistent exercise. However, watch out for the misinformation you'll get from health club advertising. This is because exercise in and of itself will do nothing for weightloss.

Research is clear about this; standard cardiovascular exercise won't make you lose weight. Sport scientists at the University of Tampa found that standard cardio exercise resulted in weightloss in the beginning, but within a few weeks the subjects stopped weightloss altogether. In fact, during the first month, standard health club cardio exercise leads to a rise in stress, a rise in cortisol levels, and more visceral fat.[5] The misinformation spewed out by the weightloss industry is dead wrong about the benefits of exercise. Researchers have found that a regular exercise program can trigger weight gain from fat, not from muscle.[6] Other studies point to one reason this is so: the more people exercise the more they initially overdo it, this then triggers cortisol and its weight gain nightmare.

Next, because of the hard work, exercisers tend to reward themselves with the wrong foods, smoothies, energy drinks, and the wrong nutritional timing. As workouts stop, hunger roars up and is often treated with a caffeinated coffee drink of some sort, loaded with sugar and milk. This instantly triggers cortisol and insulin, and here comes more fat storage.

Refuse to believe that you need a gym membership, a personal trainer, and gleaming machines to maintain your exercise level. You may feel that these provide the motivation, and if this is the case, you should join a gym. However, there is nothing keeping you from a simple exercise routine in your garage or a park that provides all of the same benefits of a gym, and you'll save huge amount of time and money.

With exercise there's a built-in acknowledgement that it doesn't burn off fat anywhere close to a balance of calories in, calories out. In that 3,500 calories equal a pound of fat, you would need to burn up 3,500 calories via exercise to weigh a pound less. So, if you ate nothing all day you would need to run six hours on a treadmill to burn 600 calories per hour, or nine hours of fast walking to burn 450 calories per hour. In this mode of thinking there is no pleasure built in, no plan of action to manipulate hormones to do the work for you. The narrative that exercise burns fat is terrible misinformation that will lead to frustration. Instead, by linking a specific exercise with an overall hormonal plan you'll be best served.

No one mentions one of the most important tools at your disposal in your effort to lose weight. Sleep. The inter-relationship of exercise and proper diet involves a real key to weightloss, sleep. Moderate regular exercise aids in sleep, especially if that exercise isn't overly intense or long. Nervous energy is a serious problem to quality of sleep, and moderate regular exercise has been clinically shown to reduce anxiety as well as sleep apnea.

Of particular interest to the Carefree system is how quality sleep maximizes nightly HGH secretions. This complex hormone is secreted by the pituitary gland in the brain and this all happens as you sleep. It is so critical to weight control, is optimally secreted in the first hour of sleep, and the more sound the sleep the better. A second and third smaller secretion comes within three hours of quality sleep, once again the amount of HGH being influenced by the quality of sleep.

Other important hormonal functions are triggered by quality sleep, especially cortisol and leptin, and the sum of these hormonal actions equals weightloss. Sleep should be at the top of the list of weightloss tools, and exercise makes for better sleep.

66 days

"I believe in everything until it's disproved."
    ~ John Lennon

Conventional wisdom tells us that it is a "fact" that it takes 21 days to develop a new habit or to break an old one. The 21 day time frame makes it sound scientific; it gets quoted over and over until it is assumed to be true. But it isn't scientific and it isn't true.

The source for this 21 day habit idea came from a popular best seller book in the 1960's by a Los Angeles plastic surgeon who wrote *Psycho-Cybernetics.* In it, Dr. Maxwell Maltz claimed to have observed that amputees took an average of 21 days to adjust to the loss of a limb. Therefore, he came up with the notion that the same must be true of all habit changes. As easy as it is to last for 21 days trying to absolutely and forever develop a new habit, there is a slight problem with this concept. It doesn't work. Research by Dr. Phillippa Lally and her collogues at University College in London helps confirm how the 21 day habit idea is a myth. Her study into how people form habits, recently published in the *European Journal of Social Psychology* turns out to be of great significance to anyone trying to lose weight.[7]

Dr. Lally's subjects, who were trying to learn new habits such as eating fruit daily or going jogging, took much longer to establish habits than 21 days. She found that the accurate number is 66 days before the behavior becomes automatic. Individuals in her study ranged widely – some took 18 days while others took 245 days – and some habits, unsurprisingly, were harder than others to make permanent.

Another myth discovered in Lally's research was the idea that when forming a new habit, you can't miss a day or all is lost.[8] The study found that missing a day made no difference. In fact, believing the 21 days in a row myth may be a serious problem for weightloss, making it harder to restart once you fall off the wagon. What Lally's study found was that the key is long term consistency, not a 21 day sprint. Therefore, it's time to rethink the dietary information you get flooded with. Physically, it is quite possible to lose 5 to 10 pounds in a week. There is no doubt that you can starve and spend significant time in the bathroom to lose 15 to 20 pounds in 20 days. Now comes the unpleasant part of the equation. Humans don't separate the physical side from the mental side. For weightloss, the result of separating the physical from the mental and emotional side will result in the classic yo-yo diet.

For you to change your life around, you need to form solid habits, and the research is clear that those habits take much longer than previously thought. Habits are reflexive actions, what we do without thinking or planning. As creatures of habit our minds and bodies are dependent on familiar patterns and actions that ultimately define who we are. The habits we develop become our security blankets that we use for comfort and familiarity. We do things unconsciously like cracking our knuckles only to find that we can't remember when this habit began but being almost incapable of breaking the habit.

This is in fact great news. If you diligently work for 66 days on changing your point of view (attitude) while you focus on a Caribbean oriented diet, and simultaneously work on regular modest exercise, you can develop the essential habits needed to lose weight. Much of what you need to do to succeed at the Carefree Caribbean Weightloss system come as a direct result of making new habits.

You can then keep it off for years by repeating the same simple program over and over, restarting every couple of months. You develop a habit of it as easily as you developed a habit of cracking your knuckles. With focus and patience, you physiologically imbed the weightloss habits that will guide you to change your life.

Let go

Finding your way to this all-important Caribbean mindset of relaxation takes work. The work can be as simple as making yourself smile dozens of times every day, starting now as you read these words. But the work must be thorough and consistent or it will just wash off without penetrating deep within you.

Nothing you can do in your weightloss efforts will help you unless you really, truly let go of the tension that binds you. The now infamous Rheingold Institute Study in 2012 sadly confirms this. This study found that modern day Germans are so stressed by responsibilities that they find it nearly impossible to let go so as to experience pure pleasure. The fear is that their "joy gene" is somehow broken.[9] Responsibility-stressed Germans have become so overwhelmed by tension that they increasingly find it hard to feel good. It's statistically worse with younger adults. Even when having sex, the study found that a broad spectrum of Germans can't focus on sex pleasure in part because they experience distracting thoughts of responsibilities rather than just forgetting everything.

The study found that one of the few things joyless Germans do tend to enjoy is jealousy directed at anyone who seems to have fun. Complaining and getting even with juvenile-like retribution was consistently cited in the Rheingold study to be a popular form of pleasure to those in the comprehensive study of 63 adults. Researchers noted that 91 percent of the subjects said that pleasure makes for a worthwhile life, however only 15 percent could remember times when they actually cleared their mind to just feel happy. Of the participants, 55 percent stated that they are increasingly unable to enjoy anything.[10]

Before you make up your mind to lose weight, you'll need to make up your mind to leave your stress behind you – a lot better than the Rheingold participants. The top of the list of things to do should be to enjoy the ride, not necessarily saving yourself for the perfect time far off in the future.

One obvious thing missing in the Rheingold study was the Caribbean sun, sand, and attitude. There the music, the sound of the waves, plus a couple of *Pina Coladas* would have had a significant wakeup call on the joy gene.

Even at home in Oklahoma during winter, it would be easy to conjure up the joy gene. Here the music of the Caribbean Islands plays an important part of changing life. Now add some interesting exercise, the aroma of a pot of Caribbean stew, some flatbread, and a glass of wine and you're in business. The joy gene will be fed and nurtured.

Four

HORMONAL FAMILY REUNION

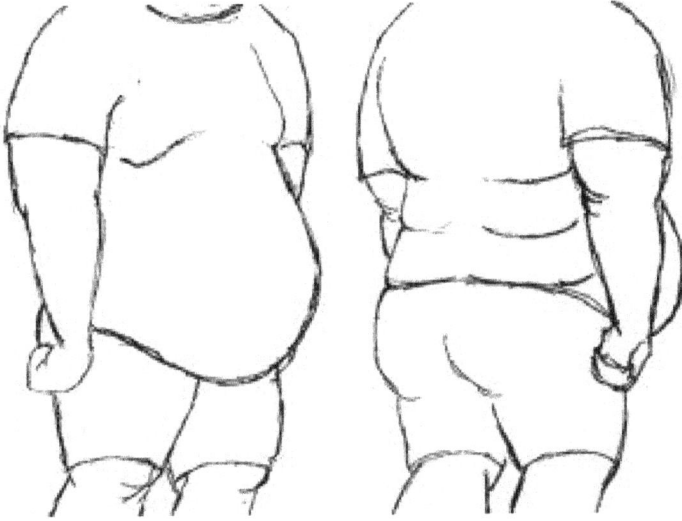

"The good thing about science is that it's true whether or not you believe in it."
~ Neil deGrasse Tyson

The people living on Caribbean shores have had it rough since the first Mesoamericans landed there around 1200 BC. With Columbus came the *conquistadores* and their descendants, through Blackbeard and the pirate era, through slavery and the Toussant Louverture era slave revolts, through the mass of Asian indentured servants, through the mixed race offspring of sugar plantation owners, through the Rough Riders, Poncho Villa, Batista and Castro…the Caribbean Islands and tropical beaches are rich with history, drama, romance and legend.

The regular hurricanes and their destruction makes this part of the world alive with a unique spirit of survival. It is fitting that the resulting culture and cuisine is so full of life, so unpretentious, so built upon rebuilding.

Another hurricane, another bout of destruction, another time to rebuild. Hurricanes are just another time to sigh and work for a better life. Troubles come, troubles go.

Despite the hurricanes, it should be no surprise that Caribbean culture has thrived through one key person: grandmother. She was the holder of family history and holder of babies. She was the cook who kept everyone alive and smiling through even the worst of times. And she was the medicine woman.

Grandmother's medicine kit consisted of herbs, roots, seeds, leaves, tree bark, flowers, and the Island chicken soup of the soul. She not only knew the foods that cured stomach ache, she knew the foods that helped children grow strong. She was the glue that held the unique Caribbean social patchwork together.

Grandmother knew that certain foods caused behavioral changes, some for better, some for worse. She knew that having lots of fish helped the health of her flock, but she didn't know that the docosahexaenoic acid (DHA) of the omega-3 fatty acids in fish was the working agent. She simply knew seafood was abundant, tasted great, made people healthy, and made her family happy at meals.

Survival was what she brought to this tumultuous land. Grandmother inherently understood that survival was a day at a time with a heart that believed things would somehow get better. There was no quick-fix, no self-pity, no prince-charming to wait for. By her attitude of persistent work and reliance on nature's bounty, grandmother made sure that her family would survive and thrive.

Nature's medicine cabinet

The entire weightloss system presented here clearly begins with an attitude adjustment similar to grandmother's. It's all about being active (exercise) and eating the right foods to manipulate your hormones. In reality, attitude and mood play key roles in manipulating hormones, thus there is a real juggling act to getting hormones to behave.

It's imperative to understand the basics of your endocrine system to have any chance at steering it to help you. You don't need to go back to college to study endocrinology, but you do need a refresher on how the system works and how to influence it.

You already know many key factors of endocrinology without thinking about it. We've all watched a room full of children go bonkers when they eat sugar, thus we all have some experience with the insulin rush. We've all experienced hunger leading to a growling stomach, thus we all know the call of ghrelin. Clearly, humans experience the effects of how certain foods cause hormonal secretions that result in observable behavior.

Our ancestors observed changes in behavior due to what they consumed, thus they knew a thing or two about balancing hormones. Without knowing what these chemical messengers are, ancient man knew the effect that certain foods had on health.

One example is the juice from olives. For 5,000 years mankind has placed high value on the fruit juice known as extra virgin olive oil, so much so that it was traded as gold. With regular but moderate consumption of olive oil, today as in the past humans can aid in balancing hormones, losing weight, and improving life all by enjoying the peppery taste of olive oil. Olive oil and other nutrients so prevalent in the Carefree weightloss system specifically target hormone reactions to metabolize body fat and to aid in relaxation.

The grand network of hormones manage bodily functions and can quite easily be manipulated by what you eat and when you eat it. After you eat and while you rest, some hormones are secreted to go to work, while others are left to wait their turn.

Hormones often signal the body to do uncalled for things. We are told to shiver when it isn't cold, to panic when there is no danger, to have a growling stomach an hour after a big meal, or to store additional fat when there is an abundance of fat. These signals can come from a multitude of reasons, from blood contamination, to psychological problems, to organ dysfunction.

It should be noted that many of these are medical problems that must be treated by a medical practitioner if a fresh food diet doesn't help. Obesity and the extreme risk that it puts on the human body needs to be addressed by a medical specialist and never delayed until it's too late. Don't put off seeing a physician as this can lead to organ failure.

Glands and organs including the adrenals, pancreas, pituitary, thyroid, ovaries, and testicles regulate most hormone production. Other hormones are produced in body fat, the brain, and the stomach. Like the instruments in a big Latin band, some blare loudly, while others are barely noticeable, but all work together in harmony. However, modern existence is so filled with synthetic toxins, industrially produced foods, and never ending stress that hormones can easily fall out of balance. The band then makes awful music.

We ruin our hormonal balance in many ways by the way we eat and the way we live. However, we also create devastating hormonal imbalance by misunderstanding. For example, we do great damage to hormonal balance by misunderstanding bacteria. Research shows that bacteria is key to gut health, and gut health is key to hormonal balance.[1]

After decades of fighting against bacteria of all kinds, of anti-bacterial food care, of anti-bacterial food storage, of anti-bacterial soap and anti-bacterial air fresheners, now the human gut shows the ill effects of all this. We've thrown out the baby with the bath water. A diet lacking basic probiotic foods to line intestinal walls can also cause hormone imbalance, triggering hunger hormones and stress hormones.

Gut care and health is of the utmost importance to weightloss. You'll need to spend time learning how the human gut functions, how this microbiome is harmed, and how it can be brought back to health. Avoiding modern synthetic toxins should be at the center of your efforts, as these toxins harm the microbiome, and a dysfunctional microbiome is devastating to the endocrine system. With a conscious effort, you'll need to eat foods that help the growth of specific gastro-intestinal (GI) bacteria to aid your weightloss efforts.

Hormonal roll call

"In the 21ˢᵗ century our tastes buds, our brain chemistry, our biochemistry, our hormones and our kitchens have been hijacked by the food industry."
~ Dr. Mark Hyman

Of the 200 hormones that make up the human body, focus on the top dozen that control weightloss; the remainder will fall in line. To lose weight you basically turn on fat burning hormones while turning off fat storage ones, all while making sure the calming hormones are happy. You do all of this by starting with an attitude of changing your life into something more fun and relaxing, but with some long-term rules. Then you eat better and live actively each day as you relax so as to not to think of the details, but to learn enough to be confident about what you do.

You select the foods that help manipulate hormones to metabolize fat and follow by avoiding the foods that manipulate hormones to store fat. For losing weight, not all produce is created equal. There are several vegetables that are vitally important, and there are several fruit favorites to avoid. This, then, is the Carefree Caribbean system.

Manipulate the following:

Adrenaline	*Emergency high-stress hormone gives instant energy, triggers fat metabolism.*
Cortisol	*Prolonged stress hormone, gives morning energy then triggers sugars into fat storage.*
Dopamine	*Triggered by pleasure and sugars, choked by hunger. Low dopamine leads to weight gain.*
Estrogen	*Female sex hormones (also affects men) triggering fat storage and binge eating.*
Ghrelin	*Hunger hormone to increase food intake and fat storage.*
HGH	*Human Growth Hormone triggers cell reproduction, regeneration and fat metabolism.*
Insulin	*Balances blood sugar, takes glucose from carbohydrates for energy and storage.*
Leptin	*Satiety hormone from fat cells, master of the metabolism.*

Progesterone	*Female sex hormone, is the opposite of estrogen, acts to burn fat.*
Serotonin	*Feel-good hormone, appetite suppressant.*
Testosterone	*Sex hormone for men and also affects women, key to metabolism.*
Thyroid	*T2, T3, T4 hormones control body temperature, metabolism, regulates body fat.*

Adrenaline

Adrenaline (epinephrine) is secreted from the adrenal glands in emergency situations, both physical and mental. It regulates heart rate and increases the volume of blood circulation while glycogen (sugars) get metabolized and sent to muscles. This is the "fight or flight" jolt of energy.

Adrenaline all by itself is an appetite suppressant. However, in times of high stress adrenaline teams with cortisol, and it is cortisol that orders you to gobble simple carbohydrates as a way to gather energy for more fight or flight. These carbohydrates then trigger insulin to send the resulting sugars to cells. Adrenaline also prepares fat for burning in this emergency. Furthermore, adrenaline metabolizes abdominal fat as it connects with fat cell receptors; these are plentiful in belly fat. For weightloss, it is obvious that adrenaline is difficult to manage.

Although you won't effectively trigger adrenaline via diet, the right exercise can help you do the job. In short burst exercise (short but intense work such as resistance training followed by a short rest) adrenaline triggers instant white-hot jolts of energy. If the exercise consists of a series of bursts about 20 seconds in duration, significantly more energy is required and significantly more fuel is burnt.

In exercise, adrenaline only gets triggered at near total output (90%+). The problem is that this level of intensity is the danger zone where most competitive sports injuries occur. In intense exercise for adults trying to lose some pounds the chances of injury are very high, especially for anyone who is over 25 years old and not in competitive sports.

The good news is that you can trigger adrenaline in certain intense exercise and not have to go to the hospital. There are several very high intensity exercises you can safely do to get fat metabolizing benefits. Push-ups are a safe and high intensity exercise, and bench pressing works as well. TRX straps (suspension cords) can be safe and effective, and heavy dumbbells offer several intense exercises without a high chance of getting injured.

Thyroid hormones

"When I was going through menopause, I didn't sleep. I didn't sleep for two years and ended up blowing out my thyroid, and I became nonfunctional. It's difficult to remain fully present if I'm not getting enough sleep, so I work at getting enough."
~ Oprah Winfrey

Manipulating thyroid hormones can make you lose weight, reduce stress, and be a lot happier. It takes no starvation, no pills, no magical juices, and no college degree in endocrinology. Start by regularly eating fresh beets and learn as much as you can about the thyroid gland.

It is quite normal to have two hormones work in tandem. When the thyroid and adrenal glands work in tandem, real bad results occur when one or the other malfunctions. When working as they should, the two act as your body's major metabolic engines. Recent clinical studies in weightloss have shown that whenever you eat less and exercise more your metabolism fights back against you by reducing energy, increasing hunger, and slowing your metabolism to a crawl. Most of this metabolic slowdown and resulting abdominal fat storage comes from the body's sensation of starvation, triggering a thyroid and adrenal malfunction.[2]

Thyroid hormones regulate the rate that you burn calories, your heart rate, body temperature, mood, and other functions. When thyroid hormones are out of balance by being too low or too high, a flurry of hormonal messages and reactions occur. If your thyroid gland doesn't make sufficient thyroid hormones, you suffer from hypothyroidism, a very common problem. You'll feel the results of this with cold hands, but all senses will be disrupted as you feel disoriented and in a fog.

The three primary thyroid hormones are T2, T3, and T4. The numbers represent the quantity of iodine molecules that are connected to the hormone. The balance and conversion of thyroid hormones must be seen as of critical importance to women for many health and weightloss problems. Low thyroid hypothyroidism can be manipulated; the first thing to do is to alter your diet. The Carefree Caribbean system of high amounts of fiber, high amounts of specific vegetables including beets, more omega-3 fats, and probiotic yogurt is a very easy way to start manipulating your thyroid hormones.

Leptin and ghrelin

Find your friend leptin and make yourself a lot thinner. Leptin's job is to balance energy between intake of fuel, expenditure of energy, and amount of fat storage. Men have twice as much leptin, so women must work twice as hard to manipulate their limited supply.

Leptin is often called the "master hormone". It signals the entire endocrine system when there is food taken in for energy and how much of that food energy should be burnt. By signaling that you're full, leptin therefore controls hunger as it teams with insulin and T3.

Although it would be great to have high levels of leptin to burn energy and shut down hunger, it isn't quite so easy. The more weight you gain, the higher level of leptin you have in circulation, but the brain becomes resistant to leptin's signaling. Too much leptin from too much body fat causes leptin resistance, where the brain doesn't respond to leptin's call. The body shouts but the brain doesn't listen.

Researchers have yet to learn all of the mechanism by which leptin regulates energy balance. However, they do know that leptin suppresses an appetite-stimulating enzyme called neuropeptide Y. Leptin also boosts metabolism to help regulate body weight by burning visceral fat for energy. The hormone is secreted from fat cells, and levels are correlated with body fat percentage. Overall, manipulating leptin is a key objective of the Carefree weightloss system.

The hunger hormone, ghrelin, is leptin's difficult relative that can ruin a good time and drive you crazy. It is also known as lenomorelin, a peptide hormone manufactured in the GI tract. When ghrelin is released it signals the brain that leptin's work is done. Then the body reacts as if there's a starvation crisis as you can actually hear the stomach growling.

Ghrelin levels are important as a marker of how soon hunger comes back after eating. Hormonal balance should trigger hunger at three hour intervals after a meal, but if you're starved after just two hours, that is ghrelin growling inside letting you know that something isn't working correctly.

Sugars trigger ghrelin and snacking on crunchy food such as carrots or celery trigger it. Salty chips instantly trigger ghrelin, stimulating you to overeat once you get your meal. Since ghrelin is triggered by chewing, clearly you should avoid chewing gum which increases hunger pangs in that critical time period from three to four hours after a meal.

Hunger signals get stronger and stronger just before you eat, then decrease soon after the meal begins, then go away for about three hours after a meal. The fourth hour is very important and this is the most difficult time as leptin shuts off and ghrelin builds up. There are many tricks to quiet the ghrelin beast. Green tea should be your first line of defense. In that vinegar quells ghrelin, many people have a salad preceding a meal with a balsamic vinegar dressing. Sleep and relaxation quell ghrelin. Balance oriented exercise effectively shuts off ghrelin.

Cortisol

Poor ol' cortisol, the most disruptive hormone of all. You need to tame cortisol in order to have any success with weightloss. Cortisol is a vitally important joint lubrication hormone that is also catabolic, reducing lean muscle mass. It's made from cholesterol in the adrenal glands located on top of each kidney. This difficult to manage hormone is normally released in response to waking up in the morning. But the problem comes when it returns uninvited due to snacking, excessive exercising and stress.

Cortisol is like a neurotic relative, always bothering you with yet another problem blown out of proportion. Excess cortisol destroys protein needed to build and maintain muscle while causing the body to store excess visceral fat. Often cortisol is referred to as the "belly fat hormone" due to its effect on the body to store more fat in the abdominal area. And worst of all, cortisol pays another unwelcome visit every time you are stressed, often following a rush of adrenalin. It is therefore of utmost importance to your efforts in weightloss that you become proactive about reducing stress, regularly doing stress reducing activities, and actively teaching yourself to have a carefree attitude so as to limit the amount of cortisol circulating within you.

Cortisol wouldn't be there if it didn't serve a purpose. The "cortisol factor" is essential to human health and well-being. This is the natural morning release of cortisol into the blood stream, typically within an hour of waking. It is associated with breakfast and the consumption of cortisol producing complex carbohydrates, then allowing the natural process of fat metabolism to take place. After letting morning cortisol go to work for you, it is time to shut down all food consumption for about four hours.

Any hunger within this time can easily be overcome with green tea. This is one of the most healthful beverages on the planet. Green tea's bioactive compounds are well known to reduce the creation of free radicals in the body, thus protecting cells from damage. The amino acid L-theanine so abundant in green tea provides moderate energy and an alert mind, just as it has for a thousand years with Buddhist monks.

Using several dietary and other tricks, you can easily dial down your stress level. Then cortisol can be of great help to your weightloss efforts. Cortisol regulates energy by selecting the right type and amount of micronutrients (carbohydrate, fat, or protein) the body needs. However, if you fail to reduce stress, cortisol will be triggered causing very negative behaviors. A stressful day can drive you to eat an entire bag of chips or a heaping bowl of ice cream, and this will set off a falling row of hormonal dominos headed in the wrong direction.

The purpose of releasing cortisol is supposed to be to give you a burst of energy in a difficult time. However, it then remains at a high level due to sustained stress, leaving you craving high simple carbohydrate snacks.

When you snack on high carbohydrate foods including energy drinks and energy bars, your blood sugar stays in the emergency zone without stop. Consistently high blood sugar levels along with insulin action lead to cells that are endlessly starved for sugar. Cells are then fed sugar in abundance for hours at a time. Multiple studies show that excess stress leads to excess cortisol, and excess cortisol leads you to accumulate abdominal fat in the hips.[3] To make matters worse, you add to stress and more cortisol by being stressed and fretting about it.

There is good news. You can take control, you can reduce stress, you can reduce your circulating cortisol level even when the pressures around seem overwhelming. Toxins raise stress, and the traditional Caribbean foods are very low in toxins and also detoxify.

Traditional Caribbean foods with their high fiber vegetation form an effective way to lower cortisol. Spinach (high in magnesium) along with a fresh garden salad reduces cortisol and hunger.[4] Throughout Latin America, chickpeas (garbanzo beans) along with other beans are eaten regularly, and these are excellent for reducing cortisol. Citrus fruits, omega-3 rich foods, zinc rich meat and shellfish are all part of traditional Caribbean meals and all aid in reducing cortisol.

The world's best chocolate is cultivated and produced on the Caribbean shores in Venezuela, and has for centuries had a medicinal effect on humans. As you read this, take a bite of dark chocolate and allow its minerals and phytonutrients to reduce your cortisol levels. Fabulous dark Caribbean chocolate is an instrumental part of the Carefree system. This isn't candy bar stuff, it is 70% cacao and higher. You'll recognize it when you taste it, and it sometimes takes a while to adjust to the strong flavor.

Yet another way to control cortisol is with exercise. Watch out, this can backfire if you don't understand how to manipulate cortisol. Hard charging exercise, go-for-the-burn routines, triathlon training, and others can easily result in more stress and the release of cortisol. A comprehensive study of over 120,000 US adults from 1986 to 2006 shows that these forms of exercise result in a quick loss or weight followed by long-term weight gain.[5]

There's more good news about manipulating cortisol, as a positive result has been found in a mixture of balance-oriented exercise and a small amount of short intense bursts. Think of this as a yoga class with a few bouts of rope climbing and push-ups. The balance oriented motions can be dance-like rhythm or circus-like balance walking.

The result of balance oriented exercise has been shown to significantly reduce blood cortisol levels, reduce adrenalin, and raise GABA, the brain calming neurotransmitter. Balance oriented exercises that emphasize proprioception (that wiggling action as you fight for balance) results in a noted improvement in mood with a reduction of anxiety, similar to yoga, according to a recent study at Boston University.[6]

For example, balance a broomstick while standing on one foot, or balance a big book on your head as you sit down and get back up. The concentration this takes aids your efforts to reduce stress while at the same time developing strength. Here is balance development, strength development, stress reduction, and hormonal manipulation in an interesting exercise that lasts a couple of minutes.

Insulin

The most well-known hormone affected by diet is insulin. Produced by the beta cells of the pancreas, insulin must be manipulated to do its job then stop; otherwise high levels of insulin induce fat storage. Although it directs how we grow and use energy, remember that insulin is medically used for weight gain for chronically underweight patients.

When left with a high amount of simple carbohydrates in the GI track, insulin goes on a binge of emergency alerts. So much insulin circulates that neuroreceptors fail to respond, and sugar gets dumped into the blood stream. This excess insulin leads to insulin resistance.

Insulin resistance is a serious medical problem. It is when there are low glucose levels in the liver and muscles, thus skyrocketing blood sugar and glucose storage. A body that has years of excessive simple carbohydrate consumption can sink into chronic insulin crisis. The pancreas produces more insulin in an effort to help glucose travel into the cells, but the result is that blood sugar jolts to catastrophic levels.

Here is where diabetes and obesity get their start. It doesn't come from excess calories, it doesn't come from excess fruit and vegetables, it doesn't come from excess fats, and it doesn't come from red meat. The problem is excess amounts of typical carbohydrates that trigger this hormonal gang fight. Carbohydrates come from a wide range of things we swallow, including sugars, starches, milk products, and yes, even fruit.

Together with leptin, insulin regulates food intake and metabolism. Performing as they should, insulin and leptin have a combined effect of suppressing appetite. Your goal each day, then, should be to help control these two hormone levels so they don't team up to harm you. With the right food and ample time between meals, you can quite easily control the insulin/leptin double team.

Being proactive with insulin levels can have life changing effect. Learning to control insulin levels by reducing the consumption of trigger foods such as sugar, common starches, and excess caffeine can help you reduce fat storage.

Even excess milk product intake stimulates insulin secretion, as dairy's unique blend of protein with carbohydrate results in a very high insulin release. A typical breakfast of caffeinated coffee with cream, cereal with milk, and a little cinnamon roll is a recipe for insulin disaster. However, the same cup of coffee with a tiny bit of honey, a bite of garbanzo bean cracker or rice, and scrambled eggs will produce the opposite effect. This is how you make the small adjustments to manipulate insulin.

The foods that bring insulin under control are all every-day Caribbean foods that eliminate insulin spikes and maximize glucagon. A diet high in clean fresh produce, high in natural fiber, high in clean protein and high in clean fat will manipulate insulin for you. You don't need to worry or over-think the insulin problem. Instead, eat a filling Caribbean meal, stay active, relax, and wait four hours until your next meal.

HGH

"The fridge had been emptied of all Dudley's favorite things – fizzy drinks and cakes, chocolate bars and burgers – and filled instead with fruit and vegetables and the sorts of things that Uncle Vernon called "rabbit food."

~ J.K. Rowling

Human growth hormone is produced naturally in your body to promote muscle growth and recovery. Importantly, HGH is essential in the breakdown of fat cells. It's found in higher concentrations in children as it is necessary for growth, however it declines with age. This decline in HGH and finding ways of getting it back into the system is the reason that it is often touted as the anti-aging hormone.

HGH has been a misunderstood hormone for many years. From its ban by sports organizations to the blatantly false advertising of yet another product supposedly elevating your HGH, it has reached the analysis to paralysis stage. No, you won't get an extra dose of it snorting a spray that claims to be made of crushed deer antlers. Yes, you can easily create an environment where your own natural HGH will be optimal.

This stuff is highly valuable for weightloss and especially for athletic performance enhancement. You can buy synthetic HGH from China, import it illegally through the mail, and inject it at your belly button. Prices range between $500 per month for the grimy street drug variety up to $5,000 per month for the supposedly clinical version. It will help you lose weight. However, there is a downside as your head will swell by two hat sizes, your hands grow much bigger, and internal organs grow similarly.

For men and women seeking to lose weight, maximizing the natural supply of HGH is essential. It is created by eating traditional Caribbean foods and living an active life. First, eat a diet high in protein, high quality fats, a high amount of vegetation. Make certain to avoid dietary synthetic toxins which have a devastating effect on HGH as well as sex hormones. Match this with a moderate amount of just the right carbohydrates as you avoid as many toxins as you can. Make sure to avoid snacking and avoid fruit juice between meals. Follow this with balance oriented exercise that includes short bursts of intense exercise. Finally, relax and sleep. The Carefree system is built upon these practices to reduce stress and manipulate HGH and other hormones.

When insulin joins with HGH, you're in for trouble as they team up and stash visceral fat. The reason is that insulin blunts the release of HGH. Therefore, your effort should be to keep insulin levels low and provide yourself with the perfect environment to maximize the release of HGH.

If for no other reason than maximizing HGH, the careful selection of carbohydrates and when they are consumed becomes instrumental. The human body needs carbohydrates and there is nothing wrong with them, despite the fad of avoiding them. Low carb diets are clearly not the way to go as there are many contraindications with the fad of low carb diets, particularly in reference to insulin resistance.[7,8] However, there is a world of difference between a low carb diet and carefully selected carbohydrates eaten at carefully selected times.

Maintaining a low insulin to high HGH ratio is surprisingly easy to manipulate. Make sure you don't eat a late dinner, ever. Give yourself a four hour respite between eating and sleeping. This is because insulin from a meal requires about three hours or so to rise and then fall. To have homeostasis at 11:00 PM means that the last food swallowed would be at 7:00 PM. After insulin subsides and you fall asleep, you'll get an optimal jolt of HGH about an hour after falling asleep and another jolt about three hours after falling asleep.

Balsamic vinegar is a great secret weapon to manipulate your HGH to the optimum while at the same time improving your insulin sensitivity. Meat and protein triggers HGH production. But this protein needs to be broken down into its component parts, the amino acids, for HGH to be made. The potent acetic acid in vinegar helps you break down protein in your meal into amino acids, as well as being a tremendous aid in absorbing minerals. Hippocrates in ancient Greece recommended vinegar for many ailments, most of it coming from "sour wine" or balsamic vinegar. For

2,000 years balsamic vinegar has been a Spanish delight made from grapes, thus its sweet and sour taste. Mixed with olive oil and seasoning, this makes a delicious "user friendly" salad dressing that also manipulates your hormones. There are many Caribbean recipes that use balsamic vinegar, each one tastes amazing.

Snacking strangles HGH secretion. In that testosterone and HGH double team for metabolizing body fat, great care should be taken to manipulate these hormones. Snacks of simple carbohydrates and even snacking on fruit elevates insulin levels to interference with HGH production, leptin production, a rise in ghrelin, and a failure to allow neuropeptide YY to effectively choke off appetite. Misinformation about snacking on so-called energy bars backfires when the net result is to dull HGH production.

Food that is particularly effective at manipulating HGH is built-in when you follow the Carefree system. The amino acids from eggs, full fat Greek yogurt, and especially seafood and meat can double HGH levels over baseline. Blueberries and blackberries help to elevate HGH. Pineapple has many benefits for weightloss, one benefit is that it aids in the release of serotonin that works as a neurotransmitter to relax brain and body, help in sleep, the perfect environment for HGH production.[9,10] Make a habit of a little desert of Greek yogurt, berries and pineapple.

Testosterone

Testosterone is essential for any man or woman who wants to lose weight, build muscle, and enjoy sex. Surprisingly, the male sex hormone testosterone is also present in women although it amounts to only 10% of the volume as in males, it is just as important. It is essential for feeling energy for men and for women.

Crash diets reduce testosterone production while obesity chokes it off completely. This is really bad because research published in *Clinical Diabetes Review* shows that low testosterone is directly linked to fat gain.[11] In fact, testosterone is so effective at burning fat that testosterone therapy is used as a treatment for obesity.

Sadly, all diets reduce testosterone. This is a key reason to avoid dieting and replace it with eating better food at better times. Diets, dieting fads, and dieting mentality are the opposite of wise, healthful living.

Instead, your goal should be to find a way to control what you eat and still maximize your testosterone secretion. A filling meal and the sensation of satiety aids in pushing testosterone levels up. This is a basic component of the Carefree Caribbean system. You need to feel full after a meal, but if this meal is made up of a high percentage of vegetation, starchy vegetation, along with quality fats in your protein, you'll trigger the "full" button without triggering the fat storage button.

A carefully managed diet and exercise program will trigger testosterone for weightloss. With an exercise program that includes short, intense bursts, the body releases lactic acid which builds up making you feel sore in your muscles. This then triggers the release of testosterone and HGH. These two hormones team up; they are two of the most powerful fat burning and muscle building hormones you have, and they have a special action metabolizing belly fat. HGH opposes the fat storing action of cortisol at the belly, while testosterone is a building block to the production of great numbers of b-receptors in belly fat. B-receptors are the locks that testosterone keys into.

Your fat cells have a variety of different receptors for different purposes. It's as if each receptor is a car and the car keys are the various hormones and neurotransmitters. When a specific key works to start a specific car, a reaction occurs. For this analogy, focus on the reactions that result in fat metabolism.

The actions of testosterone and HGH metabolize abdominal fat during exercise and also make those fat cells more susceptible to being metabolized the next exercise session. Most diets, especially crash diets, seriously lower testosterone levels and kill off the libido. Multiple clinical studies have shown that eating a typical low-fat diet instantly drops testosterone.[12] Crash diets and rapid weightloss critically elevates stress and sleep deprivation as it drives hormonal imbalance. Then the typical crash diet also has you "exercising to burn off calories."

Crash diets and rapid weightloss almost always consist of cardiovascular exercises that actually further reduce testosterone levels.[13] It gets worse. As we age the body converts testosterone into estrogen by using aromatase, the enzyme in body fat. The higher levels of estrogen slow testosterone production. The lower the testosterone, the higher the visceral fat, specifically belly fat. And so the domino effect goes, along with your growing abdominal fat and sinking ego.

Men and women absolutely must manipulate this prized hormone, testosterone. It is secreted a little or a lot, and your efforts must be to get the maximum. There's little evidence that testosterone drugs are beneficial.[14] Even if they were effective, there is zero chance for long term weightloss change if you don't significantly change your habits in terms of testosterone production and manipulation. Pills won't work. Lying in a hospital bed hooked up to an IV won't help you make lifelong changes.

You need to take charge of your own weightloss program. Therefore, it is now the time to raise your testosterone level by altering the way you live and eat. Change your diet to manipulate testosterone levels upwards and change your exercise habits to do the same. All you need to do to accomplish this is to adopt the traditional Caribbean foods and lifestyle along with your own exercise program as long as it includes a little time on balance and resistance. Then sit back and relax.

Estrogen and progesterone, a bad sibling rivalry

"Food is not just fuel. Food is about family, food is about community, food is about identity. And we nourish all those things when we eat well."
　～ Michael Pollan

Estrogen is a fat storing hormone. Progesterone is a fat burning hormone. For women, being overweight and pear shaped has little to do with calorie counting or exercise. It has a much to do with estrogen and progesterone imbalance. The good news is that you can eat to take control.

Normal estrogen levels are a biological sign that you have enough food. When estrogen signals its devious friend ghrelin to say that you are starving, your stomach growls. Then estrogen uses this an excuse to instantly create an imbalance with progesterone. Most often, people then feel starved, lazy, depressed, and helpless.

For the most part, women in their 30's see estrogen levels rise and in their 60's see the levels decline. In those three decades estrogen bullies, torments, and frustrates. In theory, the body functions perfectly and normal hormonal levels trigger satiety. In reality, as estrogen balance with progesterone gets worse, it leads to insulin resistance as the body thinks and acts as if it were starving. There is a direct effect on storing body fat.

Progesterone is the dominant female sex hormone that is the polar opposite of estrogen. It is primarily made by the ovaries at ovulation. The job of estrogen is to hormonally balance progesterone along with testosterone, but estrogen often shows up to work at the wrong time. Progesterone is the great hormone to have as a friend, responsible for romantic feelings, upbeat mood, and less body fat. It helps thyroid hormones function more efficiently, lowers insulin levels, and is a natural anti-inflammatory. Progesterone is a woman's natural sleeping pill, that is, until it is choked off by estrogen.

Body fat is a fundamental gear in the endocrine machine. It is the least understood but one of the biggest triggers of the production of estrogen. Although estrogen is also produced from the ovaries, it is the teamwork of fat plus the ovaries that produce the bulk of estrogen. Fat tissue with its aromatase converts testosterone to estrogen. Therefore, the more fat you have, the more estrogen you have. The more estrogen you have, the more fat you have.

Excess estrogen has a domino effect on people suffering from thyroid problems, slowing metabolism and adding body fat. It starts as estrogen storing excessive body fat, and that fat producing more estrogen. This rapidly turns into a vicious circle where any thyroid malfunction makes you fat and your excess fat makes your thyroid malfunction. The problem all started as estrogen, acting behind the scenes, gets other hormones to join in an evil trick on you.

Typically, women work themselves down to a plateau that is still 25 pounds too much with nearly impossible-to-remove visceral fat in the abdomen and hips. There it stays no matter how many carbs are cut or how many hours are spent in the health club. The reason is well beyond the solution of caloric balance, or the conventional wisdom of calories in, calories out.

It would be a gross oversimplification to believe that estrogen, working alone and unaided by hormonal conspirators, makes you fat all by itself. Estrogen is a part of a destructive team, that, left without intervention, will conspire to make your life miserable. When estrogen starts its hormonal domino effect, you lose. Trying to find balance between estrogen and progesterone is a 30 year war, often fought hour to hour.

Then environmental toxins enter the war; xenoestrogens from plastics, phytoestrogens from soy. The critically stressed body becomes overwhelmed and sends the problem off to the liver. But it isn't out of the body, as estrogen bullies fat cells to stay parked in the abdominal and hip region for decades.

This is truly a vicious cycle. However, the cycle can be broken by manipulating estrogen gradually downwards and a gradual loss of fat. There are no miracle foods or magical juices from the Amazon jungle that will solve the estrogen battle. But a careful selection of clean and healthful food, of finding relaxation through it all, of exercising half an hour most days of the week can help you gradually find your way back to health and happiness.

You'll get immediate help from beets. They have an abundance of betaine (trimethylglycine) which taste great and chemically bond with foreign estrogens in the liver. Little by little, betaine drags (chelates) these estrogens from the liver, leading to hormonal balance. Button mushrooms also chelate bad estrogens out and berries are great for chelating estrogens. Citrus peel, that great zest for waking yourself up in the morning, is an excellent chelator of bad estrogens. Finally, cruciferous vegetables are an every-day food to remove bad estrogens little by little.

Fibrous foods help maintain the balance of estrogen to progesterone. Research published in *Intensive Dietary Management* shows that increasing fiber consumption by 15 grams per day (which would measure to be about two avocados) significantly lowered estrogen levels in premenopausal women. The study also found that for women, a critically low carbohydrate diet can lead to estrogen dominance. The connection is clear; eat high fiber carbohydrates such as sweet potatoes in a modest amount along with fibrous starch vegetables such as winter squash and avocados to balance estrogen.[15]

For women in the midst of estrogen imbalance, vitamin B helps to manipulate your hormones and to help you lose weight. Vitamin B is necessary for the liver to break down estrogen. Foods rich in vitamin B-6 are excellent in the battle to help maintain your estrogen to progesterone balance. These foods include omega-3 rich seafood, walnuts, pumpkin seeds, poultry, pork, avocados, and spinach.

Make sure to only eat meat, poultry, and dairy that haven't been industrially loaded with additives as these can disrupt estrogen balance. Ample vitamin C is important for maintaining estrogen balance. Research has shown that 750 mg of vitamin C taken every day for six months can considerably increase progesterone production, countering estrogen dominance and its trigger for weight gain.[16] The take home message is clear; enjoy lemon, lime and grapefruit regularly.

Actively raise your mineral levels to help balance estrogen. Zinc is essential for the production of adequate levels of progesterone. It is the mineral that prompts the pituitary gland to release stimulating hormones, providing a domino effect to bring hormonal balance. Good sources of zinc come from poultry, pork, shellfish, garbanzo beans, pumpkin seeds, and dark chocolate. You also need to elevate your magnesium intake to help to balance estrogen. Get more magnesium by eating spinach, plantains, pumpkin seeds and yet another bite of dark chocolate.

Be certain to maximize vitamin D in the effort to manage estrogen. Vitamin D isn't just a vitamin; it's a precursor to a steroid hormone. It is a strong source of balancing hormone levels, particularly estrogen. Get more vitamin D by going out into the mid-day sun and walk for a while, enjoy the sun and relax. Vitamin D is also abundant in salmon, sardines, yogurt, eggs, oysters, pumpkin seeds, coconut, spinach, garlic, and cruciferous vegetables. Every one of these food choices is an integral part of the Carefree Caribbean weightloss system.

Feel-good hormones

Sin and enjoy it.

Overcoming stress is at the very heart of the Carefree Caribbean Weightloss system. Stress will negate all you do to lose weight; therefore you need to effectively overcome stress. It must be done, it can be done, it is done all the time. Food all by itself won't overcome the stress that makes life so unhappy and makes weightloss so difficult. You need to manipulate hormones that are made for the job of reducing stress. The starting place is an attitude adjustment. After that comes a carefree but active life with rules about what is consumed and when.

To be successful with the Carefree weightloss system you need to make a great effort to actually be carefree. Concentrated work should be done every day, several times per day on being happy. There are simple actions you need to do that proactively help overcome stress and allow you to be happy. There is a great drug for this and it is inside you now as you read these lines, just waiting to be released and make you smile. In fact, just the act of smiling right now will start the process of feel-good hormone secretion.

Maximizing feel-good hormones shouldn't be left to chance; they need to be grown like a favorite plant. Overcoming stress is vital to weightloss, much more important than a list of rules posted on the refrigerator.

Sipping wine, enjoying *Pina Coladas*, or enjoying a *mojito* with Caribbean rum runs counter to virtually every dietary guide in existence. But overcoming stress, having a good time with friends, enjoying the music and dancing a little – this is far more important than dietary rules. Overcoming stress comes first, way ahead of what comes second.

Next comes consciously manipulating hormones by diet and activity. Far after that comes calorie counting. After all, Caribbean life as we know it would vanish without the devil rum.

The human body has several anti-stress hormones including serotonin, dopamine, endorphins, and oxytocin. These not only make you feel great, they add an effective tool to your weightloss efforts. Feel-good hormones are your mood regulators that make you tranquil, focused, emotionally stable and calmly energetic.

Much of the triggering of feel-good hormones comes from habits and attitudes. For example, dopamine is the human "motivation hormone" that is choked off by self-doubt and procrastination. Here is a case where your attitude and behavior manipulates hormones, either positively or negatively. Those who doubt that attitude has a direct effect on weight gain need only study and experiment with the way that dopamine can be physically turned off and on almost like a light switch.

Feel-good hormones make life worth living. Serotonin brings a drug-like glow; it's produced by nerve cells and results from eating certain protein but it only enters the brain with carbohydrates as well. Dopamine gives feelings of being mentally alert and is triggered by eating protein rich foods. Endorphins reduce anxiety, reduce sensitivity to pain, and come after a session of intense exercise. Oxytocin brings a glow of love and trust; it comes from the pituitary gland during emotional and passionate times.

Each feel-good hormone is appetite suppressing and erases stress as it relaxes. Each one feels pretty damn good when it hits the brain.

Serotonin causes an overwhelming sensation of a good mood, sex desire, memory and learning, that "warm glow" temperature regulation, and is great for cool and calm social behavior. As a byproduct, it aids in digestion. But for weightloss, serotonin is essential because it eliminates all stress, anxiety, fear, bad memories, self-doubt and irritation from barking dogs. It is part of your endocrine system, it is safe, and it can be manipulated.

Serotonin is manufactured from the tryptophan you get from specific foods, some good, some not very good for you. Here is the start of the problematic food-mood connection in life. There is no direct food source of serotonin, but there is for tryptophan. Foods high in protein, iron, and vitamin B6 all tend to contain large amounts of tryptophan. The problems come from the carbohydrate delivery service to the brain which tend to be the most counterproductive carbohydrates because the drive for them is directed by passion.

Tryptophan rich foods don't necessarily increase serotonin on their own because the tryptophan must compete with other amino acids to be absorbed into the brain. The body turns to simple fast-acting carbohydrates as a substitute. Then as you excessively chomp a plate of cookies, insulin levels go through the roof. Insulin triggers the absorption of amino acids and the tryptophan levels rise. The brain gets its beloved tryptophan but the body gets visceral fat.

The way to manipulate the system is to find tryptophan rich foods that can be eaten as part of a meal. Protein that is rich in tryptophan should always be eaten with fat and a little of just the right carbohydrates.

Manipulating hormones with food from the Caribbean

Once again, Carefree Caribbean nutrients do the job for you. For example, whole eggs, so prevalent in Caribbean recipes, are protein rich and raise blood tryptophan. As long as they come with dietary fats (this means the whole egg, not just the whites) and a little resistant starch, they are an excellent hormone manipulating tool to pass the blood brain barrier. This is a way to describe the standard Caribbean breakfast of eggs cooked in coconut oil along with roasted yuca "fingers" along with a bite of pineapple. There are many other tryptophan friendly foods found in Caribbean cuisine.

Bromelain-rich pineapples are a great tryptophan source of carbohydrate, along with sweet potatoes. Mushrooms, Wild Alaska salmon, shellfish, pork, poultry, and Greek yogurt are all rich in tryptophan. Each of these food items optimally result in getting serotonin in the brain.

Garbanzo beans and dried bean flour form one of the truly great complex carbohydrates that are regularly consumed in Caribbean meals. Because they're taken up slowly and steadily by your body, they have a stabilizing effect on your blood sugar and your mood, keeping you energized and raising tryptophan so as to elevate your serotonin. You don't need a lot, just a handful regularly sprinkled on your salad and regularly making garbanzo bean flour flatbread (*faina*). This delicious garbanzo bean flatbread should become a staple for anyone seeking to lose weight.

Eat folate-rich asparagus and spinach to manipulate the tryptophan to serotonin process. Your brain uses the B vitamins in these foods to make serotonin along with multiple other functions of weightloss. The enemy of serotonin is cortisol. The higher the cortisol levels, the lower the serotonin. It turns out that sleep is the key to which one wins. Getting enough sleep is mandatory to choke off cortisol and allow serotonin to flow freely. A recent study in the *Journal of Clinical Neurology* found that cortisol levels can rise significantly after a single sleepless night.[17] Thus you need to take great care with sleeping well so as to manipulate serotonin as a way to lose weight and live better.

Sunlight and exercise provide the environment needed for the production of serotonin. The opposite comes from soft drinks, energy drinks, sugar, candy, and bakery items that flood you with insulin, all of which suppress serotonin. A little bit of coffee can actually help if it puts you into a positive "can do" frame of mind but be sure that coffee is only consumed early in the day or you risk triggering cortisol.

Clearly, serotonin is way up on the list of hormones you need to optimize if you wish to succeed at long term weightloss. With its regulatory ability to affect mood, social behavior, digestion, sleep, memory, sexual desire, sexual function, and appetite, serotonin is critically important to manipulate. Your brain makes serotonin and serotonin makes you happy. A happy you is a person with low cortisol. A happy you is a confident you that you can succeed at long term weightloss.

Serotonin is so important to manipulate that it is known as the "don't worry, be happy" hormone. Of importance to weightloss is the way that exercise and serotonin work together, as the right stress-free exercise boosts serotonin in the brain. You can increase your serotonin in your system by regular exercise.

Carbohydrates such as bread, potatoes, pasta, pastries, pretzels, popcorn, play a big role in the serotonin puzzle. These foods increase insulin which then open the gates for tryptophan to convert to serotonin. Within about 30 minutes there is a calming sensation as you enter your happy time. However the blood sugar rise causes multiple problems followed by the classic drop in blood sugar and the filling of fat cells.

Once again, Caribbean agriculture and dietary habits save you. Great taste and long term complex carbohydrates such as sweet potatoes, garbanzo beans, carrots, and even blueberries boost serotonin without the corresponding drop in blood sugar that comes from bakery goods and simple carbohydrates.

Gurgling hormones of passion

Oxytocin is a hormone you need in abundance, preferably several jolts each day. Oxytocin is released by the hypothammus in the brain and then into the bloodstream by the pituitary gland. This hormone is hopelessly misunderstood by the weightloss world and should be considered as essential.

It is a hormone released by feelings of love and trust, by wild sex and by petting your dog. Not only is it part of the orgasm sensation, it shuts down appetite until love subsides. For men it is released with an orgasm in times of love and trust, not necessarily with a casual sex partner.

Oxytocin floods the body when women are in labor and women get a jolt of it during breast feeding, a time of tremendous weight maintenance for so many women. So this hormone clearly doesn't act alone out of some bottle to make you thin.

This strange hormone is not very well understood by scientists, complicated by the fact that it is released in abundance watching tearful movies and also from shooting guns, though not necessarily at the same time. Snake oil salesmen rush to the opportunity to bottle it and sell it but reality gets into the way. Although oxytocin can be purchased as a nasal spray (Syntocinon), there is no evidence it works.[18]

Oxytocin is triggered when other hormonal factors are working, blended with other feel-good hormones. This hormone regulates food intake even though certain foods trigger it. Those foods are mostly associated with love and passion, so it is difficult to determine if it is the food itself or the mood of the meal that triggers oxytocin.[19] But this is the wrong way to think of this wonder hormone. If asparagus and oysters trigger it, go for it. If you just *think* that asparagus and oysters trigger the passion in you, go for it. This is because the mood of love triggers the hormone of love.

Proactive hormonal help

Behavior that triggers feel-good hormones:

Laugh more, turn chuckles into full-fledged belly laughs.
Take a long, deep breath frequently each day.
Take a bath, or a dip in the lake, or a swim in the surf.
Hug your pet, rub his head, scratch her ears.
Do balance oriented exercise often.
Smell the roses, really.
Walk in the sunshine.
Go barefoot, wiggle your toes often.

Food that triggers feel-good hormones:

Avocados	Almonds, cashews
Asparagus	Beans
Beets	Garbanzos (chickpeas)
Dark chocolate	Eggs
Peppers	Salmon
Spinach	Sweet potatoes
...and maybe oysters	

Five

FEED YOUR HORMONES

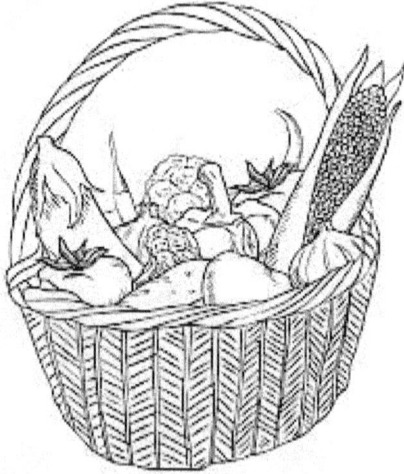

"Let food be thy medicine and medicine be thy food."
~ Hippocrates

The quality of what you eat plays a critical role in your weight. Food tells hormones what to do, and hormones make people fat or thin depending on the type and quality of food as well as timing of meals. Our entire endocrine system is so interlocking that as one hormone triggers it signals another to fire which triggers another and so on. Virtually all hormones regularly do multi-tasking and double teaming.

These chemical messengers secreted into the bloodstream by endocrine glands and other systems can be our best friend or worst enemy. Although complicated to understand at first, it's not difficult to learn how to manipulate them to fire so they help lose weight. No doubt it'll be surprising to learn that many of the things thought to be of help in weightloss actually cause hormones to work against us.

By not taking control, by failing to be observant, we blindly eat the wrong foods that trigger hormones to do the wrong things to the body. To make matters worse, we eat the right foods that have been contaminated by the wrong toxins and this results in the wrong actions. And then there is stress; we live in a stress-filled life and even exercise in a way the body reads as stress, telling hormones to store fat. To solve the issue, we adopt yet another hopeless diet and exercise program which only makes things worse. Living in this chaos is a recipe for staying fat.

With much fanfare, Oprah Winfrey announced that she loves bread, that bread is part of her life and her heritage. In spite of overwhelming evidence pointing to commercial bread as a primary hormonal trigger for maintaining body fat, she made a choice to continue eating bread.

Not a word was said about how modern industrial refined grains lead to visceral fat. No comment on the takeover of industrially designed stunt wheat from the wholesome wheat that mankind has eaten for millennia. Nothing was spoken about the standard 37 chemical additives in commercial bread.[1] Oprah then stated that to counter her love of bread she joined Weight Watchers. The volatile combination of commercial bread plus Weight Watchers calorie counting will ensure that Oprah's choice will most likely result in a never ending yo-yo diet.[2]

Twenty years ago, Weight Watchers created their point system to count calories. In essence, this started a weightloss company that profits over $180 million per year by getting people to just count calories regardless of the food integrity of their boxes of chips and powders they sell. The result has been to get people to spend more money to rapidly lose weight only to see initial weightloss turn into weight gain. There are literally dozens of other weightloss programs modeled after the calorie counting concept.

As for buying clean fresh food and preparing it at home rather than buying mass marketed processed meals and drinks – this can't compete. Unfortunately, fresh home cooked meals don't have multi-million dollar advertising horsepower to make them popular. What we do buy to be prepared for home is then mixed with boxes and jars of industrial sauces and condiments brimming with synthetic chemicals and toxins.

Standing in the grocery store checkout line it is amazing to look at what's in the other grocery carts. People spend so much money on jugs of Coke or Gatorade or other brightly colored sugar water mixes. You'll see boxes of processed foods, carts sprinkled with packaged artificially flavored chips or sweet treats. Cans and jars of condiments and sauces are randomly thrown into the cart. Regardless of the calorie count, the quality is terrible. The cost of these low nutrient industrial foods far exceeds the amount paid for meat and eggs. A rule of thumb is that at least half of the money spent on "food" in grocery stores goes to buy empty calories and processed carbohydrates that cause so much damage to health and the weight problem of the nation.

Make your change by becoming manipulative

"In a chronically leaking boat, energy devoted to changing vessels is more productive than energy devoted to patching leaks."
   ~ Warren Buffett

Change. Take control. Once you carefully choose what you eat, you select via hormones the signals you want to send to your brain and body. Those signals are then sent to your organs to perform prescribed tasks to get the body to burn white visceral fat, the evil empire of obesity.

To take control of your endocrine system, you have to give up those foods and behaviors which harm you, and happily adopt new foods and behaviors that help you. Just the comfort of your solemn decision, the relaxation it will bring, and the sense of satisfaction will trigger hormonal change, delivering more serotonin and less cortisol to help in your effort to metabolize visceral fat. Athletes call this, "relax and win."

Hormones are produced in a body environment of good fats and cholesterol. Fats make hormones work. The lack of these important nutrients causes hormone malfunction simply because the body doesn't have the building blocks to make sufficient hormones without dietary fats. Here is an example of misinformation telling you to only eat low fat foods, avoid egg yolks, and use spray cooking oil with harmful industrially made hydrogenated fats. This will manipulate hormones the wrong way. You trigger more visceral fat storage by eating "heart-healthy" egg-white-only omelets and low-fat yogurt because of insufficient quality fats which feed the desired hormones.

Leptin is produced in fat cells, and upon release into the bloodstream it goes to the brain to say that you've had enough food, you've reached satiety. As you get hungry and snack several times per day, even snacking on fruit, you halt the release of leptin which could, were it not interrupted, function as a day-long regulator of energy balance. When leptin is present, it metabolizes fat for energy. Once the leptin signal in interrupted, ghrelin is released and you get ravenously hungry, halt the fat burning process, and go crazy until you eat again.

Choose carbohydrates very carefully, as these have a key hormonal effect. The one-two punch of excess insulin and cortisol comes from a high carbohydrate diet, leading to having ghrelin overwhelm you with hunger. If you drink coffee in the afternoon, you trigger the release of cortisol and adrenalin to team up, stimulate your adrenal glands, and this daily overstimulation leads to adrenal failure. Here comes belly fat storage.

By the wrong food choices and the wrong time to eat, you fail to let leptin do its job. Misinformation plays a key role here. All of us are told to snack on low fat processed turkey slices, whole grain bread, russet potatoes, commercial spinach, snacks with processed egg whites, and worst of all, soy. In this way, the entire weightloss industry of doctors, nurses, dietitians, nutritionists all tell you in effect to interfere with leptin/ghrelin control. The very thing that makes people fat comes at the suggestion of the very people who are supposed to help you lose weight.

Hormone manipulation for weightloss takes planning. First, remove as much toxin (petroleum fertilizer, herbicide, fungicide, preservatives, artificial flavor, artificial color, emulsifiers, and artificial taste enhancers) from your diet as possible. Then eat a clean produce dominated diet with emphasis on a large amount of fresh vegetables and a small amount of select fresh fruit. Eat free-range animal protein, eat sufficient dietary fat early in the day, and avoid snacking for four hours after each meal. Go to bed four hours after dinner and ingest nothing between dinner and bed that would interrupt the hormonal process. This will help take control of the endocrine process. Repeat this most days and nights of the week.

Fresh produce plays a major role in hormone manipulation. Regularly eating high fiber vegetation acts to decrease estrogen levels, decrease cortisol levels, and stabilize blood sugar. There are several produce items to pay particular attention to. Regularly enjoy beets to trigger adrenal and thyroid hormones as this greatly enhances fat metabolism. Broccoli and cabbage should be eaten most days of the week to help towards estrogen balance. Raw vegetables are vitally important for their unspoiled load of phytonutrients, and you get them in a green salad (with spinach or beet leaves replacing lettuce) to raise your magnesium levels in order to reduce cortisol. With the right flavor, you'll love this change.

Caribbean meat dishes are typically made with a mixture of vegetables and flavored with herbs and spices. These spices not only flavor the food but provide excellent hormonal manipulation. Start with much more garlic and a broad variety of onions. Black pepper, turmeric, cinnamon, basil, and cayenne help to manipulate insulin to convert glucose into cellular energy before it is turned into fat storage. If you can tolerate heat, enjoy hot Jamaican jerk to bring water to your eyes and flood you with endorphins to tame cortisol. Gradually adapt yourself to the sizzling wonders of Central American and Mexican hot, hot dishes.

Sprinkle hormone manipulators to your dish. Fresh pineapple, especially the core, is high in bromelain which stimulates the release of HGH and serotonin. Beans (red, black, garbanzo, fava) are high in L-dopa which stimulates the pituitary gland to circulate more HGH. A small amount of protein rich Greek yogurt on top of a dish or mixed with berries for desert not only adds flavor but raises HGH production.

Although leptin levels aren't raised directly from foods, you can manipulate the environment for optimal leptin function by raising dietary zinc simply by sprinkling nuts on your salad or using pumpkin as you would use potato. There is a long Latin American tradition of eating mineral-rich dried pumpkin seeds (papitas) for a treat.

Manipulative tricks

"A foolish consistency is the hobgoblin of little minds, adored by little statesmen and philosophers and divines."
Ralph Waldo Emerson

Let yourself go, break away from harmful habits. You can easily manipulate your nighttime hormones by being careful before bed. However, if you are careless about your sleep you won't put yourself in a state of deep sleep which will bring the optimum hormonal release.

Turn off all ambient light so you basically sleep in a cave. If necessary, get black inner curtains for windows to block out street lights. Make sure to cover miscellaneous lights (battery recharger lights, smoke detection lights, computer router lights, etc.). There are nutrients to help you sleep better including magnesium, calcium, melatonin, and Vitamin B.

When you wake, start in on hormone manipulation. Get up and immediately head to the kitchen for grapefruit, lemons or limes. With a zester or a knife, put your nose right next to the skin and sniff a little of the spray from the peel. These floating droplets of citrus spray trigger dopamine, serotonin, oxytocin and endorphins. All of this action is because the liver produces more enzymes when stimulated by citrus than by any other food source.[3]

Immediately slice the citrus fruit in half and drink the juice. The bioflavonoids (antioxidants) will have instant results on improving insulin resistance by regulating glucose down and providing the environment to raise leptin. Fresh squeezed citrus juice elevates alkaline levels, and research indicates that those with the highest alkaline levels tend to more effectively lose weight.[4]

Whatever you do, don't fall for the myth of thinking that a glass of orange juice, even fresh squeezed orange juice might help. This will do nothing positive for weightloss, as processed orange juice is actually orange flavored sugar water with a bit of vitamins added. This is in fact a major contributor to weight gain.

Next you enter the coffee-yes, coffee-no argument. There are two schools of thought on this. The coffee-yes argument is that due to high antioxidant and polyphenol levels, coffee jolts you awake to think and act, cranking up the metabolism. The coffee-no argument is that it puts stress on the liver, leads to adrenal fatigue, and causes anxiety. Then there is the coffee-companions argument, that the stuff we swallow in coffee or nibble along with coffee is worse than the coffee itself.

The shores of the Caribbean Sea produce the world's greatest coffee, arguably Costa Rica produces the best there is. Coffee is a major part of the history of this land and its people, it is consumed by the ton there, and the smell of it brewing in a Caribbean café is stunning. Cuban coffee is a ritual to make, from beans to a pinch of sugar whisked to a foam. Coffee is more than just coffee bean juice, it is part of Caribbean blood.

If there are two sides to the coffee argument, tradition wins here. Fresh brewed coffee is part of the lifeblood of the land and therefore something to be sipped in moderation first thing in the morning, but only in the morning or you trigger cortisol later in the day. To succeed in this Carefree Caribbean journey, you need to take part in the culture, the heartbeat of the land, and coffee is part of the Caribbean soul. Coffee, rum, and dark chocolate make the world a better place, help you enjoy life, and are woven into the fabric of Caribbean life.

Coffee alerts us all to timing. One thing that has shown to have very consistent weightloss result is the clock on the wall. Pay attention to nutritional timing and see the results last for months, even years. Gaze at the clock daily, watch the calendar weekly. The 6 days on, 1 day off routine works very well. Be diligent for six days and weigh yourself on the morning of the 7th day. Then you are free.

This is a tremendous psychological relief valve that is simultaneously a hormonal relief valve. This weekly off-day serves several hormonal purposes, surprisingly similar to re-booting your computer to flush out the system. Shock your hormonal system to get out of neural fatigue in order to become more sensitive to signaling. Enjoy the foods you have so strictly avoided, but never let in environmental toxins or preservatives.

Your off day can have lots of forbidden fruit carbohydrates and calories, but absolutely not synthetic toxins. Off days are your devil rum days of debauchery.

Kitchen hormonal therapy

Eat to lose weight. You only need a few bites of this and a spoonful of that, but the cumulative effect is to take charge of your hormones. There are many food choices to manipulate hormonal response and they are right in front of you at your nearest grocery store. Here's a start.

Animal protein: *Glycine rich foods, meat, dairy (yogurt or hard cheese) raise HGH and control insulin.*

Asparagus: *Anti-inflammatory, rich in B vitamins, magnesium, zinc, and potassium. Balances estrogen.*

Avocado: *Antioxidant, anti-estrogenic, raises testosterone in men and progesterone in women.*

Beets: *Betaine detoxifies liver, chelates xenoestrogens, and builds testosterone and HGH.*

Berries: *Flavonoids in berries help balance thyroid hormones so essential to metabolism. Highly anti-inflammatory.*

Garbanzo beans: *High zinc stops aromatase, converter of testosterone changing to estrogen, helps balance estrogen to progesterone.*

Citrus: *Grapefruit, lemons and limes are highly alkaline and increase HGH. High in antioxidants improve insulin resistance by regulating glucose and leptin.*

Coconut oil: *High in magnesium and vitamin B12, aids adrenal function and thyroid health. Very quick energy and hunger suppressant.*

Cruciferous vegetables: *Alkalize gut to raise HGH, reduce estrogen, detoxify liver. Broccoli, cauliflower, cabbage, kale.*

Dark chocolate: *Highest plant magnesium source, high tryptophan helps raise serotonin, oxytocin, HGH, reduces cortisol.*

Eggs: *Choline and iodine in yolks balance thyroid hormones, raise testosterone. Lower insulin, ghrelin, while raising peptide PYY.*

Fats:	*Focus on more omega-3 fats, meat and seafood top the list. Virgin olive oil, dairy fats, egg yolks, all raise testosterone, lower estrogen, release leptin.*
Fiber foods:	*Avocados, cruciferous veggies, sweet potatoes reduce estrogen levels. Lignin fiber in beans helps stabilize blood sugar, fat, and estrogen levels.*
Garlic:	*Garlic's sulfur compounds and diallyl disulfide (most active when crushed) will trigger more testosterone.*
Green tea:	*Blocks cortisol release, extends norepinephrine release, helps block release of ghrelin via enzyme CYY to ensure optimal carbohydrate metabolism.*
Leafy greens:	*Mix of spinach, kale, arugula, romaine lettuce, beet leaf volume extends sensation of satiety; the fiber provides environment for maximizing leptin.*
Mushrooms:	*Mushroom variety helps to reduce estrogen, rich in vitamin D to maximize testosterone production. Treats adrenal fatigue.*
Nuts:	*Rich in amino acid L-arginine to stimulate HGH. Highest Omega-3 and best hormone balancing nuts are almonds, Brazil nuts, walnuts.*
Omega-3 fats:	*Sardines, anchovies, cold water fish for leptin sensitivity, serotonin environment elevated in brain. Eggs, beef, and beans also good source.*
Papaya:	*Carotenoids in papaya are a hormone balancer that tend to reduce anxiety and mood swings.*
Pineapple:	*Best taken at dinner, muscle relaxant that helps release of melatonin and environment for serotonin to stimulate HGH. Acts as sleep aid.*
Pumpkin:	*High in zinc and magnesium, aids progesterone release to balance estrogen. Seeds are anti-inflammatory, help conversion of LA to GLA omega-3 fats.*
Red pepper:	*Red bell peppers and red hot peppers rich in antioxidants and vitamin C, curbs cortisol.*
Red wine:	*Resveratrol in red wine aids glucose uptake to help control insulin and aids in balancing hormones. Can aid in release of oxytocin.*

Resistant starch: *Aids in conversion of tryptophan into serotonin in brain. Stimulates digestive enzymes that stall release of ghrelin.*

Sea salt: *Helps adrenal function, high in magnesium and many trace minerals that aid thyroid function.*

Sweet potatoes: *Rich in vitamin A to maximize testosterone and the environment for serotonin release. Positive effect on estrogen balance.*

Vinegar: *Balsamic vinegar lowers blood sugar, curbs release of ghrelin, aids insulin sensitivity. Cook with small amounts of apple cider vinegar.*

Yogurt: *Careful, organic only and high protein, full fat. Probiotic which balances hormones. High protein aids production of numerous hormones.*

Foods to avoid

Avoid these foods. Be very careful not to be fooled by the misinformation of food labels. Read the label word for word, but go straight to the ingredients list. Beware as official looking lists can hide harmful ingredients, too. Know what you eat. Look it up in advance so you don't get tricked at the grocery store.

Cooking Oil: *Canola, vegetable oil, safflower oil, corn oil, soybean oil, margarine, partially hydrogenated oils, shortening, all trans fats. Never use spray cooking oils.*

Dairy: *No more cereal and milk, or cream for coffee. No frozen yogurt, ice cream, sour cream. Get milk out of the house be very selective about all dairy.*

Grains: *Avoid refined grains, whole grains, bread, bakery goods, cakes, cookies, pasta, muffins, bagels, cereal, pancakes.*

Jelly and jam: *At 65% sugar content, often high fructose corn syrup (HFCS), guaranteed to raise insulin. High heat for preservation destroys active nutrients.*

Ketchup: *Very high in HFCS or sugar. Typically have "natural flavoring" which is actually taste enhancing chemical compounds including MSG.*

Orange juice:	*Basically sugar water with some added vitamin C powder and a few drops of orange flavor.*
Mayonnaise:	*Often made with trans fats, even olive oil mayo quite bad. Highly processed egg yolks from industrial hens, extremely high in preservatives.*
Processed cheese:	*Avoid American cheese, nacho cheese, Velveeta. Very limited choice of mozzarella or soft cheese.*
Salad dressing:	*Nothing processed, especially no low-fat dressing, no good-health dressing. Blue cheese and Caesar dressing particularly loaded with toxins.*
Soy:	*In almost all processed foods. Phytoestrogen that mimics estrogen triggering fat storage, interrupts thyroid function and hormone balance.*
Sugar:	*Avoid sugar, high fructose corn syrup, milk chocolate, soft drinks, fruit juice, Gatorade, Muscle Milk, milkshakes, smoothies, protein shakes.*
Sweet fruit:	*Fruit sugar (fructose, glucose, and sucrose) is still sugar. Watermelon, cantaloupe very high sugars; bananas, oranges so-so. Best sweetener is unfiltered honey.*
White potatoes:	*Very high glycemic load and farmed in very high toxic environment of pesticides and preservatives. Most potatoes (russet) eaten are highly processed.*

Starches are other fattening habits

"Conformity is the jailer of freedom and the enemy of growth."
    ~ John F. Kennedy

Conformity makes you fat. Now is the time to give up bad habits that leads to abdominal fat. The starches that you grew up on, that call out to you, that entice you with their aroma... these are criminals that make you fat. Find it in yourself to replace them, to gradually change your starch love to Caribbean resistant starches. Know what evil lurks within breads, buns, muffins, cakes, crackers, and other beloved bakery items.

In order to understand the role of starch carbohydrates in your diet, it's best to use the glycemic load (GL). It is a realistic way of measuring the relative sugar content of food. This is a ratio of the glycemic index (GI) and also portion size. The GL range is 10 = low, 15 = medium, and 20+ = high. For example, a small bowl of standard white rice has a GL of 20, quite similar to pasta. A bran muffin has a GL of 149 while a serving of carrots has a GL of 4. A high GL meal jolts insulin up, but a meal with starchy vegetables or resistant starches doesn't. If you don't know the GL of a particular food, don't worry. Stick with Caribbean tradition that has fed healthy and happy people for centuries.

Simple carbohydrates and their rapid digestion trigger a powerful insulin jolt putting you into hormonal hell. Any quantity exceeding the bare minimum necessary to keep you functioning starts a hormonal domino effect heading the wrong way. Selecting just the right nutrient packed carbohydrates to fit into a very small space is no easy task. In reality, selecting carbohydrates can be a real difficult problem.

After sugar, grains are the most problematic carbohydrate choice. With one third of the diet being made up of vitally needed carbohydrates, and that carbohydrate portion broken down into vegetables, fruit, resistant starches, beans, yogurt, a bit of honey, some red wine, and a little dark chocolate – you aren't left with much room for grains.

When you eat grains, they elbow-out the most beneficial carbohydrates that do the most beneficial hormonal work for you. Grains take up a lot of badly needed space and don't give much back in return. Wheat, corn, and rice come with a high GL, while broccoli, carrots, pumpkin, squash, and resistant starches offer much more nutrient with less glycemic load. Quinoa sits in the middle as an occasional starch, nutrient packed but also boasting a high GL.

Modern commercial wheat is the ruination of weight loss. The triggering of insulin from industrial stunt wheat is automatic. Humans react to modern wheat the same way they do to candy because of the rapid breakdown wheat and wheat products such as breads, buns, cakes, cookies, croutons, crackers, muffins, pancakes, pasta, cereal, etc. It isn't simply that wheat comes from a chemically modified plant. Bakery products are a delivery mechanism bringing huge amounts of sugar and high fructose corn syrup (HFCS), along with dozens of chemical additives, plus the worst commercial oils.[5] The glutens, the toxins used to grow the plant, more toxins to prepare it, and still more to preserve it make wheat something to strictly avoid.

After wheat, the next modern dietary nightmare is soy. According to the US Department of Agriculture, 93% of soy in the United States is genetically modified (GMO). In published animal studies, GMO soybeans lead to reproductive hormonal problems. Other studies found that GMO soy caused damage to the liver along with toxemia. High allergic reactions are directly associated with GMO soy consumption.[6] Soy is a huge crop covering 91 million acres in the US, controlled by huge industrial agricultural firms that use huge amounts of herbicides, specifically glyphosate, to produce huge crop volume. Glyphosate is an endocrine disrupting chemical that has been found to have severe effects on kidney function. It is used extensively on soy.

Almost every packaged SAD product has soy in it, but soy brings way too many problems to even be considered as a choice of food of anyone seeking to lose weight. The lectin properties in soy interfere with leptin hormonal function and sensitivity, with the result leading to visceral fat. The dangerously high phytate levels in soy bind to magnesium, zinc, calcium, and iron making these vital weightloss minerals unavailable.

Hormonally it is the soy plant-estrogens in the form of isoflavones which effectively raise estrogen levels and therefore lower progesterone and testosterone levels. Since these hormones compete with one another, more of one results in less in another. A Canadian research team found that the disruption that soy does to estrogen balance leading it to have a direct effect on visceral fat for both men and women.[7]

Cornmeal is yet another carbohydrate that is filled with too many problems to fit within the tiny carbohydrate allotment you have. Carbohydrate dense corn chips, tortillas, tamales, and other products made from cornmeal work against your efforts. 88% of corn grown in the United States is GMO, and multiple studies link GMO corn to hormonal imbalance and dysfunction. In 2012, Kaiser Permanente, the nation's largest healthcare organization, issued a warning on consumption of GMO corn.[8] The toxins in the fertilizer, pesticides, preservatives, and packaging make cornmeal an endocrine disruptor, and cornmeal is everywhere in processed foods. Recent published studies link high levels of cornmeal intake to significantly elevated estrogen levels, and estrogen dominance is a leading cause of weight gain.[9]

The good news is that a small percentage of corn is non-GMO, has a relatively low pesticide load, and it is our basic corn-on-the cob found in local grocery stores. Sweet corn has a long tradition in Caribbean dietary history, and it is an important component in the Carefree Caribbean Weightloss system.

Rice is a staple throughout Latin America. There is a Latin American slogan, "A dinner is not a dinner without rice." It's still a grain, still has a relatively high GL, but it is for the most part just rice. Very little industrial development has happened to the common grain of rice. However, rice easily fits into the Carefree system as it is typically served with lots of vegetables, tasty fish, chicken, or pork, and a handful of rice. With only a tiny slot on your plate for starch carbohydrates, those seeking weightloss should find that a small serving of rice fits into the occasional category.

Beans and weightloss

There is an amazing aroma from a pot of Caribbean beans slowly cooking all day. Beans with onions are common in Caribbean cuisine, as much a part of the meal as friendship and laughter. But beyond the smell, taste, and tradition, there is an underlying science of what beans do for humans.

Beans (legumes) are seed pod plants instrumental for any wise weightloss system, but need to be eaten in moderation, a few small servings each week. They provide tremendous nutritional benefits, aid in hormone manipulation, and their fiber is a great aid to slow down the digestive process for weightloss.

Most beans have a moderate glycemic load. However, they are often prepared in concentrated forms (baked beans, refried beans, hummus) these should be eaten in small amounts to fit into the small carbohydrate allotment you have. Be careful to avoid canned beans which come with nightmarish hydrogenated lard, preservatives, and often di-sodium EDTA just to keep them colorful.

The Caribbean way of preparation is much more nutritious and, as always, flavorful. Islanders soak them overnight then slow cook all day with onion and flavorings, which equates to tossing pre-soaked beans into a crock pot in the morning and enjoying them for dinner.

Beans have a long history of providing nutrients to Islanders, especially when eaten with corn to form a low level protein. The extraordinary mineral content of beans results in an important hormonal action, triggering HGH and testosterone. Studies have linked beans with helping to protect against inflammation, something critically important for weightloss.[10] One way they help prevent weight gain is that they make you eat less since fiber expands in the digestive tract, soaking up water and taking up high volume. Beans make you feel full in no time.

Garbanzo beans are especially important for keeping blood sugar level normal. They have a very long history of cultivation in the region. There are many Caribbean dishes featuring garbanzos, often sprinkled on top of another dish as garnishment, and garbanzo bean flour makes the greatest simple flatbread known to mankind (faina). Dark beans (navy or black) are highly alkaline thus create the environment optimal for the release of leptin. Due to their hormone manipulation capabilities, high fiber, high mineral content, beans should be considered essential, a top priority food.

Thyroid manipulation on a plate

Thyroid health, weightloss, and a great crunchy taste are all available at your grocery store. These vegetables have multiple benefits; you'll find many reasons for them beyond their unique aid to thyroid function. Conventional wisdom warns against eating cruciferous vegetables such as broccoli and cabbage because they might damage the thyroid gland. The theory goes like this: broccoli has glucosinolates that could interfere with the absorption of iodine leading to thyroid dysfunction.

Conversely, research by Christina Bosetti and other clinical studies disagree.[11] The rumor is far from the truth, as it would take eating broccoli and cabbage all day, every day in amounts impossible to digest to have any negative effect on the thyroid gland.[12]

Service your thyroid gland most days with a small amount of broccoli, cabbage, or kale. The thyroid is thermoregulatory, meaning its job is to control body temperature among several other tasks. Many people suffer from thyroid dysfunction and the results are almost guaranteed to add to visceral fat. Since a well-tuned thyroid gland is instrumental in your efforts for weightloss, aim to eat coleslaw or a broccoli stir fry or just bits of kale mixed into your salad. Carefree Caribbean eating and lifestyle should be your medicine to fight for thyroid gland health, and there are dozens of recipes to enjoy cruciferous vegetables in order to help you in your quest.

By eating intelligently, moderately, and focusing on relaxation in daily life, you can get your thyroid to perform optimally. Caribbean cuisine is made for the job of manipulating thyroid hormones in your favor. The following foods are excellent to help your thyroid function.

Almonds	Avocado
Berries	Broccoli
Cauliflower	Eggs
Green, leafy vegetables	Mushrooms
Nuts	Seafood rich in omega-3
Sweet potatoes	Yogurt

Triggering leptin

Put yourself in the right biochemical environment so that what you eat can have an impact on leptin release. Manipulating your leptin/ghrelin ratio is as easy as having sardines on garbanzo *faina* flatbread or cassava crackers. The omega-3 fats, minerals, plus the protein will regulate your biochemical levels so as to manipulate leptin and other hormones for several hours. There is no food source of leptin, clearly there is no leptin pill to take. But your efforts to create the internal environment that maximizes leptin release is easily found in your nearest grocery store.

Leptin's release can be halted or cut short by the wrong foods, starting with excessive carbohydrate consumption. The worst food choice for manipulating leptin comes from grains and sugars. Even eating at the wrong time stunts leptin, as habitual snacking between meals halts leptin and replaces it with ghrelin. Excessive stress, excessive exercise and insufficient quality sleep stunts your leptin release. Processed foods tend to cause inflammation, choking off leptin. These same processed foods clearly stimulate overeating and this further reduces leptin's effect.

The digestive tract can't absorb leptin. Since it is a hormone that is manufactured in fat tissue, clearly you need to eat foods that create the right fat environment for leptin to maximize. But it is a temperamental hormone that fails to perform if too much body weight or too much body fat is present. Therefore, it is of extreme importance for you to eat the right fats, the right fiber, and to be moderately active without having excess stress to create the right environment for maximum leptin.

Regularly eat green leafy vegetables and fiber-rich foods, as they can help keep your body feeling full, avoiding the situations that choke off leptin – specifically, snacks and stress. Leafy greens stimulate the digestive tract and keep your leptin sensitive. A produce-rich diet should be considered the motor that keeps leptin in circulation.

Nutritional timing plays a big part in manipulating leptin. Eat protein and fats early in the day to bring satiety so you don't feel starved in the afternoon. As you recall, the sensation of hunger is connected to the sensation of stress, and the two work in tandem to kill off leptin circulation. Always have a few bites of produce early in the day to get the antioxidants to reduce inflammation as you create the right environment for leptin release. A great way to accomplish this is to have grapefruit in the morning.

For optimal leptin release, you need protein along with your mandatory produce. Whole eggs, meat, nuts, Greek yogurt work towards leptin sensitivity in a positive environment. Along with protein, Caribbean high fiber avocados and coconut offer a great source of fats. Taking fish oil in the morning is a good way to make sure you raise your levels of fats for leptin release and leptin sensitivity. A nice side effect of fish oil is that 2000 mg of it daily reduces your cortisol level.

Olive oil for weightloss

"Except for the vine, there is no plant which bears a fruit of as great importance as the olive."
　　　~ Pilny

Figuring out how to eat the right fats in the right way is no easy task. You're told to remove the skin of chicken and cut off excess fats of beef or pork. You're told to use cooking spray oil made of Canola oil, nitrous oxide, dimethyl silicone and artificial flavors. Then you're told to take additional fish oil, coconut oil, and fatty vegetables such as avocados. It's easy to get confused. The best way to get through the fat confusion is to focus on high quality traditional foods. Animals that walk and eat in fields have fed humanity since we began walking on two feet. Coconuts, avocados, and olives are nature's bounty of fatty foods that have served Mesoamericans for hundreds of years.

On the other side there are many modern animal fats that are quite problematic due to the many chemicals consumed by animals and thus consumed by us. Fresh fish can be terrible for weightloss if the fish have absorbed pollutants. Skin free chicken breasts with herbs…this sounds great until you realize that the chicks are brimming with antibiotics.

The worst cooking fats such as soy, corn, and sunflower oil are quite dangerous polyunsaturated fatty acids (PUFA), entirely omega-6, and heavily treated with synthetic chemicals. Standard industrial butter is a terrible choice in fats, not because of the saturated fats, but due to the high quantity of omega-6 fatty acids and the fact that the cows are fed on GMO grains.

Olive oil comes to the rescue. Cold pressed extra virgin olive oil has generation after generation of service to mankind, in a large part due to being part of our ancestral medicine chest. It is essential for cooking, but also for skin care, hair care, reduces inflammation, stress relief, improves mood swings, earache treatment, and even helps battle heart disease. The grand tradition, the cultural connection, and the peer reviewed scientific recommendations for consuming olive oil fits perfectly into the Carefree Caribbean Weightloss system.

The juice squeezed from olives was of great value to ancient Mediterranean cultures. It became interwoven with Spanish culture, was the choice of Spanish cooking as well as preserving foods. Olive oil and olive trees that traveled to the New World with Columbus were planted within months of the arrival of the *conquistadores*. Large olive fields were planted in Argentina and Chile by the early 1500's and by 1524 Franciscan missionaries planted olives in Old California.

Columbus and early colonizers mixed Spanish foods with native Caribbean Taino tribal foods including corn, beans, squash, roots, and colorful native crops. Over the centuries that followed, olive oil was the medium that blended traditional Mediterranean foods with indigenous foods and the endless international foods brought in by trading ships. But for the most part, in the New World olive oil was an imported delicacy for the aristocrats. It took centuries for olive oil become something for the masses.

The monosaturated fatty acids of olives essentially allow hormones to stick to cell walls keeping cell receptor sites functioning optimally. This ancient oil has a direct hormonal effect, as research by Amin Derouiche has discovered that olive oil consumption brings a 17.4% improvement on testosterone levels.[13] Maintaining hormonal balance is of the utmost importance to those seeking to lose weight, and this balance is helped by a "good bottle" of olive oil. It's hard to figure out what is good and what is an overpriced goo with a pretty label. Research has found that California olive oils rank well at the top of quality cold pressed extra virgin oil.

One very simple benefit of olive oil is that the fats make you feel full, and this satiety helps manipulate the reduction of stress hormones. By regularly having olive oil and other quality fats, you actively control your insulin levels. Research published in 2010 found that in a two month study, a diet with plentiful quality olive oil resulted in more weightloss than a low-fat diet. Centuries of consumption of olive oil has built the intuitive knowledge that it improves memory and ability to focus, and these observations have been clinically found to be true. In that low-fat diets are typically linked to more anxiety and depression, a diet with plentiful olive oil is perfect for raising spirits due to its influence on elevating dopamine and serotonin.[14, 15]

Olive oil has 30 different phenolic compounds which have the unique ability to reduce oxidative stress. This is the source of the amazing anti-inflammatory nature of olive oil. It is highly resistant to oxidative damage inside you and inside your sauté pan. Cooking over moderate heat but avoiding high heat with olive oil prepares food to be tender and tasty, all while providing you with a high amount of anti-oxidants.

Sauté with olive oil and garlic. Sauté salmon and shellfish including muscles, octopus, and squid regularly. Caribbean culture makes this easy with fabulous shellfish *paella*. Seafood and olive oil mix perfectly.

Although fresh shellfish is best, frozen shellfish is highly rated by the Environmental Working Group (EWG). Most grocery stores have free range or organic meats including chicken, beef, pork, and even buffalo. Always seek free range eggs. And then cook with cold pressed extra virgin olive oil to regularly get quality fats in a diet that is so critical to weightloss. This is the Carefree Caribbean system.

How quality fats help weightloss

"In Framingham, Massachusetts, the more saturated fat one ate, the more cholesterol one ate, the more calories one ate, the lower people's serum cholesterol...we found that the people who ate the most cholesterol, ate the most saturated fat, ate the most calories weighed the least and were the most physically active."
~ William Castelli MD, Director of the Framingham Study

Since the declaration of war on fats in the 1960's, a verbal and economic battle has been waged against fats and especially against cholesterol. In no time it became a "red scare" as millions of people became obsessed with the terrible evil of fats without knowing anything about them. These carbon, hydrogen, and oxygen atomic compounds so integral in human existence somehow became demonized to the point of public mania.

In this red scare, even the most basic fats, the monounsaturated fats found in olives, nuts, and avocados became something to avoid. By focusing on the 160 calories in half an avocado, including 15 grams of fat, nutrition specialists and dietitians saw the fats but didn't see what the fats do. In fact, it is the monosaturated fats in avocado that are responsible for reducing low-density lipoprotein (LDL), the "bad" cholesterol. Furthermore, the very high anti-oxidant levels of avocados have been shown to raise metabolism, reduce metabolic syndrome, and burn visceral fat. Multiple studies have shown that avocado consumption leads to a reduced body mass index and reduced waist circumference.

After all the millions of dollars spent on pre-workout energy boosters, the lowly avocado has been found to out-energize test subjects by 13% more than commercial drinks and energy bars. This is the same fruit that has nourished an entire region of the globe for 3,000 years.

In our fat phobia, the polyunsaturated fats found in eggs, olive oil, fish, walnuts, and garbanzo beans were guilty by association, thus more reason to eat processed food. We never heard the discussion of essential fatty acids (omega-3 and omega-6), those fats that humans can't make and have to get them from our food. But we heard plenty about the glory of margarine, that chemistry project butter replacement that was low fat (horary!) but also high in partially hydrogenated fats, better known as trans fats. As the trans fats came into our diet, weight gain followed suit.

Balanced thinking and balanced health

"I don't think there's been any major shift in the medical profession's general approach to new ideas. I don't think there ever will be that kind of wholesale change. Three hundred years ago, when the major disease was smallpox, Sir Thomas Sydenham developed a new treatment that reduced the death rate from about 50 percent to 1 or 2 percent. His reward was being challenged to a duel."

~ Abram Hoffer, MD

By the 1970's as the communist red scare morphed into the fat scare, a generation of people switched from healthful fats to industrial fats. Fatty acids went critically out of balance as a direct result. We began to consume vast amounts of omega-6 fats and precious few omega-3 fats. The omega-6 fatty acids come from corn and other grains. For thousands of years, mankind got along just fine because grass fed livestock and fish (high in omega-3) balanced our omega-6 intake.

As we switched to industrial farming, livestock began to be fed all corn and soy. The chicken breasts we're supposed to eat (watch out for the fat!) became all grain fed. And the advertising mantra was that corn fed livestock were somehow better than ol' Bessie munching hay in the field. We actually sought to buy "marbled" fat beef so loaded up from corn that it was enormously fat when compared to grass fed livestock.

Within a few years, humans went from a balance in essential fatty acids to an imbalance of approximately 20 parts of omega-6 to one part omega-3 today. We eat this way because the goliaths such as Tyson foods produce 35 million chicks, nearly 500,00 pigs and 130,000 beef carcasses for us to eat every week, all made up of omega-6 fatty acids. Therefore, by continuing to follow the low-fat narrative today, we're stuck with an extremely out-of-balance diet. And as a result of our fatty acid imbalance, we continue to throw our hormones out of balance. And we get fatter.

Quality fats in the diet tell the hypothalamus in the brain to release hormones, including leptin. This is why it is a must to have daily consumption of high quality fats. Because modern industrial farming has changed our dietary fat consumption from traditional omega-3 dominance to overwhelmingly omega-6 dominance, you need to make a great effort to consume omega-3 fat foods (free range meat, eggs, full-fat yogurt, fatty fish) in an attempt to bring balance.

Rather than investigate our new fatty acid imbalance as a root cause of health problems and weight gain, nutrition specialists and dietitians said it was the fault of red meat. The red scare continues to this day, but it is fatty red meat that is the enemy. Not a word about fat imbalance.

Let the sun shine into your life

Find a way to balance food and enjoyment of the little things in life. It can be as easy as walking in the sun. Vitamin D is a hormone and you don't get it in a pill nor in a jug of milk. It comes from the sun; the same way Islanders have soaked it in for 3,000 years.

Once again there is the health argument of sunshine-yes or sunshine-no. It has benefits and problematic effects on human health. But limited exposure of walking leisurely in the sunshine would clearly be to the healthful side. Dermatologists are dead wrong when they claim that there is no safe exposure to the sun. What they are overlooking is the tectonic shift in mankind with the electrification of the planet. We spend our lives indoors and this indoor life plays a big part in our failure to move around in the sun. By moving indoors we have divorced ourselves from the multiple benefits of a leisurely stroll outdoors soaking in Vitamin D. It's relaxing, it's wonderful socially, it's excellent exercise, it's brain stimulating, and it helps quell the hormonal beasts within us.

There are tremendous benefits of going outdoors in the sunshine. Sun exposure protects against inflammation and even lowers blood pressure. The serotonin release is immediate, cued by specific areas of the retina, as the brain is programmed to relax in the sunshine. The calmness that follows lingers into the night as sleep is aided. Each of these benefits fits into the overall goal of manipulating hormones in your favor in the grand plan for weightloss.

If the day is hot or if it is cold, go outside in the sunshine, even if this means walking around an office building a couple of times. Let the sun shine on your skin and help you relax, as a vast number of neurosensors connect with ancestral past. No sunscreen please. Have you looked what's in that stuff? Be an Islander, soak in vitamin D, and enjoy walking a few minutes to unload stress. And try to walk barefoot a little each day as part of your vitamin D experience, even if it is in your back yard.

It's no coincidence that sunshine and the sea shore have an immediate effect on human romantic behavior. Multiple studies as well as empirical evidence show that the first days of a holiday in the sand and the sun equates to an overwhelming romantic flush. Vitamin D plays its part here.

Your goal as a human is to find more balance in your life. Balance in what you do, balance in what you eat, balance in how you move. It is balance, called homeostasis, that preserves mankind. Balance means eating enough to have a fully satisfying life that keeps you healthy and happy. Imbalance is to eat too much or to starve and be unhappy about it. Eat enough then stop, put enough food on your plate to eat enough then don't eat more. Excess calories are a part of the weightloss puzzle, but nowhere near the most important part. Balance starts with thinking in a balanced way.

A drinking problem

"In other words, the science itself makes clear that hormones, enzymes, and growth factors regulate our fat tissue, just as they do everything else in the human body, and that we do not get fat because we overeat; we get fat because the carbohydrates in our diet make us fat. The science tells us that obesity is ultimately the result of hormonal imbalance, not a caloric one – specifically, the stimulation of insulin secretion caused by eating easily digestible, carbohydrate-rich foods: refined carbohydrates, including flour and cereal grains, starchy vegetables such as potatoes, and sugars, like sucrose (table sugar) and high-fructose corn syrup. These carbohydrates literally make us fat, and by driving us to accumulate fat, they make us hungrier and they make us sedentary. This is the fundamental reality of why we fatten, and if we're to get lean and stay lean we'll have to understand and accept it, and perhaps more important, our doctors are going to have to understand and acknowledge it, too.
    ~ Gary Taubes

Today perhaps the most common loss of balance is in the crazy excesses of drinking. There are soft drinks, energy drinks, sport drinks, fruit drinks, smoothie drinks, along with bottled coffee and sugar drinks. These make up an enormous carbohydrate glut that has thrown us all way out of hormonal balance.[16] These endless drinks throw the endocrine system out of control and fat storage is the result.

Imagine how hard the body must work to digest Caribbean pork stew with plantains and carrots along with a garden fresh salad. Compare that to drinking a machine-made liquid that does all the work for you.

We have a huge selection to choose from: Gatorade, PowerAde, Vitamin Water, Muscle Milk, Frozen Cokes, Mountain Dew, Red Bull, 5-Hour Energy, Starbucks Refreshers, Monster, Rock Star, and countless more.

Traditional Caribbean cuisine never had industrial energy drinks and never suffered from the ill effects. In the past, they never had to think about it. The traditional Caribbean life was just to work hard and celebrate with a simple delicious fresh meal. Drinking beer, wine, and the devil rum was left for nights of fun and also nights of debauchery.

As the SAD enters the Caribbean Islands today bringing obesity and health devastation along with it, it is drinking these ever present soft drinks that play such a big role in declining health. There is no doubt that excess alcohol consumption has had a bad effect on Caribbean society as it has on virtually every society on earth. However, the drinking problem was never anywhere near the CDC calculation of 69% overweight and obese percentage of society faced today. Part of that overweight and obese tragedy rests with the modern obsession with soft drinks, energy drinks, health drinks and the like.

Don't get suckered into the drinking problem. Buy your own fresh food. Turn on some loud music, preferably Caribbean sounds. Chop your food up, cook it with whatever seasoning you have on hand, serve it up casually, and enjoy every bit of it. Thoroughly savor a piece of dark Caribbean chocolate. Rub your full stomach and relax, sip a little red wine, the same liquid that so pleased our ancestors.

This is how to adopt Caribbean simplicity to manipulate your hormones. What we choose to eat manipulates hormones, and the things we don't eat is also a choice in hormone manipulation.

Six

FOOD FIGHT

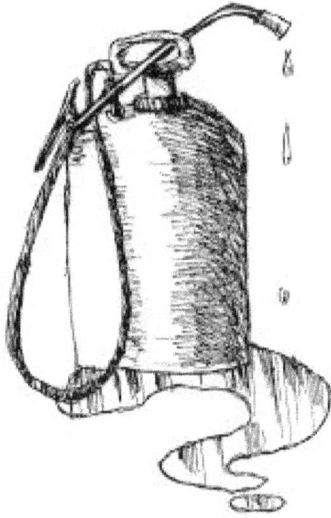

"I beseech you, in the bowels of Christ; think it possible you may be mistaken."
~ Oliver Cromwell

As much as the Caribbean Sea offers hope for all seeking weightloss, toxins can rob that hope from us. Toxins are part of modern life today in the Caribbean as in all modern societies. However, they have not become institutionalized in the Caribbean anywhere near the way they have to us farther north. It is still quite easy to find traditional Caribbean life with very low levels of toxins, but you have to know what to look for and what to avoid.

Unfortunately, it is much more difficult to navigate your way around environmental and food toxins in the United States. As you'll see in Chapter 10, many standard grocery store foods included in the Carefree Caribbean Weightloss system are considered safe by the EWG. Others are only available online at specialty stores. You can follow this guide in order to know what to get and where to find it.

The ease of careful shopping can rid you of almost all destructive toxins. However, buying anything that just looks good will do the opposite. Learn what helps you and what harms you, but don't let this become another analysis to paralysis episode. Find out what to avoid and load up on those foods that will manipulate your hormones to aid you.

Recently the EWG found 20 different pesticides on one strawberry sample. In comparison, pineapple, so interwoven with Caribbean society and diet, has very low toxin rating, provides considerably more health benefits than industrial strawberries, and can be found in almost every grocery store in America. In a screaming food fight, pineapples win.

In a similar way, it's quite easy to find meat with very low levels of toxin. Despite the extremely high amount of antibiotics fed to industrial American livestock, once you learn how to shop locally you can buy organic meat at your nearby grocery store or at a nearby farmer's market. While half the world's seafood comes from highly toxic fish farms, you can easily buy safe fish and frozen shellfish at your grocery store in order to prepare fabulous Caribbean seafood meals.

Unlike the SAD, the traditional Caribbean diet of local produce, local seafood, locally raised meat, and the lack of industrial farming means they generally consume foods with very low toxicity. The region doesn't have a significant portion of their population suffering from the ill effects of industrial toxins, either as consumers or as farm workers.

Sadly, industrially made toxins as well as residue from coal fired power plants and transportation emissions all wind up in what we eat, including in the Caribbean today. Therefore, the goal is to find the most traditional and least toxin tainted Caribbean life and cuisine to model our northern life after.

Don't let the fear of toxins or the science of weightloss scare you away. This is a fairly straightforward body of information that will help you understand what these toxins are, where they are found, how to avoid them. By finding out how to shop for the lowest toxin foods, you can pretty easily reduce toxin intake, reduce weight and live carefree.

Toxicology: the truth hurts

"I'm not upset that you lied to me, I'm upset that from now on I can't believe you."
~ Friedrich Nietzsche

There is a fascinating development in the science of weightloss that has nothing to do with calories, carbohydrates, omega-3 fats, or some magical powder. It's time to look at the science of toxicology, a new frontier of weightloss. Toxicology has unlocked the door for us all to better understand how our food industry has affected the modern crisis of obesity and a chronically overweight society. Toxicologists help us learn how synthetic toxins are part of the SAD and cause us to gain weight no matter what the micronutrients are or how many calories we consume.

We all consume synthetic toxins at an astounding rate, then we listen to industry and government soothsayers tell us that the toxins aren't really so bad. We eat toxins, cook with them, put them on our skin, and 45 million Americans continue to smoke them, according to the CDC.

For decades the tobacco industry lied about the danger of cigarettes and for decades they got away with it. Now there are multiple lawsuits charging the tobacco industry of knowingly promoting tobacco addiction.

Today the opioid crisis is directly tied to the pharmaceutical industry pushing Oxycontin onto the populace all the while industry-hired medical doctors proclaimed the safety and non-addictive nature of Oxycontin. The result is that today opioids kill more Americans than cars, thus now would be a good time to change the way to think about what government and industry tells us all about the safety of the toxins in our diet.

Studies have recently found that man-made toxins do in fact cause weight gain and diabetes. Once ingested, these chemicals alter the body's balancing act between blood sugar and dietary fats, gradually leading to insulin resistance.[1] Weight is gained, then toxins are stored for years in white fat cells around the abdomen and hips. Like zombies, these toxins want out. So we oblige them with our counterproductive diet, generational exercise mania, and crash diets.

Toxic buildup in your body is stored in fat cells. The toxins leak out or pour out and then you feel irritable. It's as if you have a hangover. This part of consuming toxins is difficult to separate the physical from the mental aftereffects. People report feeling insecure, run down, suffer from headaches, as if catching a cold. Constipation, bad breath, sensitivity to scents, skin rashes, muscle aches, constant fatigue and frustration (once again) about inability to lose weight. With all of this, millions of people turn to a crash diet to solve everything.

Crash diets are worse than no diet at all

Throughout the Carefree Caribbean Weightloss system you'll see an emphasis placed on slow or gradual loss of weight. There are sound reasons for this and toxicology heads the list. Clearly it takes an attitude adjustment to accept gradual loss of pounds while everywhere you look there are rapid weightloss diets.

By gradually losing about a pound most weeks you avoid dumping toxins into the bloodstream that overtake the human filtering system. Eaten a little at a time, you allow the right foods to clean away the most of the toxic debris. By taking your time to gradually lose weight, the toxins are therefore controlled without overwhelming you in toxic shock, pain, discomfort, depression, anxiety, and a mental fog.

A lifetime of ingesting toxins has stored most of them in your fat cells. As you go on a crash diet, many of the toxins are flushed back into the system; people often report feeling dazed, stressed, suffer from sore joints, and even feel poisoned.[2]

Crash diets are easy to start; it's thrilling to lose 10 to 20 pounds in the first few weeks. After that it's time of the plateau, where no weight is lost despite tremendous effort at dieting. This is where the circulating toxins almost take over your life. People report feeling much better when they break with their diet and eat a lot of carbohydrates, thus taking the circulating toxins out of their blood and storing them back into fat. Here is the biochemical response similar to the withdrawal of a drug addict.

When you rapidly lose weight, the toxins released into the body can feel like you've swallowed rat poison. Go on to any well-advertised crash diet, lose weight quickly, but an invisible toxic force commands you to eat more of the wrong foods to stop the pain. Is it a psychological pull back to the wrong foods? Is it a physiological pull? Regardless of the cause, the reality is an overwhelming magnetic pull away from the diet. This is a toxicologist's description of the yo-yo diet.

If you don't start out weightloss with a gradual program to detoxify you'll never permanently lose weight and change your shape due to the emotional and psychological nightmare of detoxification. This is because rapid weightloss starts with the basic formula: body fat is a protective mechanism to store toxins. However, no matter how much you exercise or how few calories you ingest, the toxins must leave the body in order for long term change can happen.

The diet industry loves this because the detoxification process has become something new to sell. Instead of having you eat lots of salad and fresh produce, the diet industry tries to sell you another product or service. The good news is that the day you begin the Carefree Weightloss system is the first day you'll detox. A year later, you'll still have lots of salad and produce and continue to gradually detox. The process won't change. It is what Islanders do without knowing that they are forever detoxifying. They eat the foods grandmother makes not realizing that they are on a detoxification program.

The human filtering system

Humans are born to detox. We evolved taking in good nutrients and bad toxins. Over millions of years, the body developed an effective system to filter and remove toxins. What we consume gets broken down in the gut and nutrients are shuffled off to various locations for further work. Most of the unwanted toxins get sent out as solid and liquid waste, others come out as sweat or breath. But the worst of the toxins stay.

The heavy work of toxic removal is done by the liver, the primary filtering system of the human body. Overflow toxins are sent to the kidneys to be eliminated. Everything has pretty much gone according to plan eliminating toxins until the arrival of man-made chemicals. They screw up the whole delicately balanced filtering system. The vast majority of toxins are our own body chemicals which act upon plant or animal invading contaminants. These powerful biochemicals such as naturally occurring free radicals are used to break down different substances into energy. Once inside, the good nutrients are broken down into usable energy, with concentrated toxins left over, ready to be removed. Toxins of all types are then selectively channeled to be kicked out of the body like some obnoxious drunk at a bar.

The liver: *The liver detoxification starts the process as it changes the chemical nature of many toxins, then sends them to exit or to stay at storage points.*

The kidneys: *The kidneys detoxify by secreting natural toxins or filtering toxins out of the blood into urine.*

The GI system: *The GI and digestive systems eliminate most food toxins, others are sent to be reworked or stored for later use.*

The lungs: *The lungs detoxify through our breath by removing gasses, including gas anesthetics.*

The skin: *The skin detoxifies with sweat, removing unwanted substances that are sent through the lymph system and circulating blood.*

In terms of volume, the liver is an enormous detoxifying factory. It cleans toxins and waste from the blood, separating the useful from the bad. Among numerous duties, the liver sends unwanted substances away, including the worst concentrated toxins in the body. Whatever the liver can't handle, it sends off to the kidneys, via bile, and back to the small intestine to be tossed out.

Another big part of our filtering process is the lymphatic system, a water filtering method to remove toxins. Lymph is a fluid with infection-fighting white blood cells needed to tame many toxins. The lymphatic system prevents debris from getting in the way and slowly poisoning tissue. This system is all connected to lymph nodes (found in tonsils, adenoids, spleen and thymus) which do the dirty work of filtering. Unwanted substances are then channeled from the lymph system to the kidneys for elimination.

Daily emptying of your lymph system occurs naturally. There are things you can do to make it work better and many of these are part of the Carefree Caribbean system. Through bouncing type exercise (skipping or jumping rope, etc.), drinking green tea with a squeeze of lime, eating select tropical fruit with your meal, and actively reducing stress in life, you can greatly aid your lymph system eliminate toxins.

The kidneys filter all blood 20 times per day

Ingested toxins are of two kinds: water-soluble and fat-soluble. Most water-soluble toxins are easily flushed out of the body via the blood and kidneys, but the fat-soluble toxins are difficult to remove.

The most dangerous fat soluble toxins include heavy metals, pesticides, preservatives, food additives, pollutants, plastic chemical residue and other man-made chemicals in the environment. They must be converted by the liver into water-soluble form for the body to fully eliminate them. If your digestive and detoxification systems aren't functioning properly, these toxins find their way from the liver to the blood, fat cells, and the brain, where they can be stored for years, setting you up for a future of serious health and weightloss problems.

Some of the stubborn toxins entering the body get lodged in organs, altering the way the organ functions. Most go through the filtering process and get shuttled to fat cells, either making more fat cells for deposit or filling up existing ones. When these fat cells are eventually burnt as fuel, the exhaust from the process is the stored toxin, back again to wreak havoc.

Toxins that hide in abdominal fat cells have to be handled carefully or they emerge at midnight like ghosts to mingle in the blood serum. Alarmingly, multiple studies have linked weight gain to elevated toxins in blood serum. One recent study by Eva Morales and her team of researchers was published in *Environmental Health Perspectives*. The research team discovered that babies were twice as likely to be obese at age six if they were born with high levels of pesticides.[3] This is a serious problem showing that many pesticides go in but don't go out, ever.

By consuming commonly eaten Caribbean foods you can aid the filtering process. For example, fresh cilantro is a widely used herb for flavor in many Caribbean dishes, especially tasty when sprinkled on hot soup. However, cilantro is a chelating food that draws out various toxins so the body can eliminate them. Toxins that get by the preliminary filtering process need food such as cilantro to bond with molecules in the various toxins. The body can then eliminate this bond.

In this way, you gradually manipulate toxins to work their way back into the kidneys, then pass as urine. The process is slow and takes place month after month, but it is progress. Caribbean attitude adjustment then comes to the rescue, as relaxed patience is the key to long term detoxification, just as it is the key to long term weightloss.

Caribbean foods tend to be very high in fiber, great for the detoxifying process. As fiber passes through the GI tract, it scrapes the intestinal walls, the microbiome which is lined with trillions of microscopic flora. These living finger-like organisms play an indispensable role in detoxification. The flora must be fed with pro-biotics (abundant in the traditional Caribbean diet) and cared for with ample water and fibrous foods to stimulate their function and growth. The microbiome flora can then perform many essential dietary tasks including playing their part in detoxification. We feed and care for gut flora; the gut flora cleans our GI tract for free. Perfect symbiosis.

As mankind evolved, this gut flora symbiosis worked without problems. We ate the foods that we had around us and adapted to our surroundings. As the islands of the Caribbean became populated thousands of years ago, people found food that worked great for health and detoxification.

Mesoamericans feasted on fish, poultry, avocado, corn, beans, roots, squash, legumes, tropical fruit, with an endless supply of local vegetation. With Columbus, the foods from Europe, the Mediterranean, Asia, and Africa were added to the bill of fare. All served Caribbean filtering and detoxification wonderfully. These fresh and natural foods worked perfectly 500 years ago and work perfectly now, except for one modern problem. Man-made toxins.

The truth, the whole truth, and anything but the truth

"All right everyone, line up alphabetically according to your height."

~ Casey Stengel

How do we get ourselves into situations of making major decisions based upon completely illogical, unfounded, crazy information? We take people at their word as we fail to spend any time looking deeper into what we are supposed to decide upon. We avoid the truth and get preoccupied with lining up the chairs on the Titanic, oblivious to the approaching disaster.

Modern dietary experts who claim to save us from the ravages of obesity and our weight gain epidemic add to the problem. For instance, Dr. Arthur Agatston's popular *South Beach Diet*, although it sold millions of copies, turns out to be a stew of misleading information.[4]

This 2003 media splash preached low carbohydrate intake, but the "good carbs" were processed breads and pasta. The good *South Beach Diet* protein was fish (not a word about what kind of fish or the relative mercury toxicity) and commercial dairy (not a word about toxins or added hormones). Nowhere did this diet warn that synthetic toxins trigger hormonal after-effects that lock fat to the abdomen. The book even encourages consuming the modern health nightmare of artificial sweeteners to reduce calories. These harm many biological functions including interfering with weightloss.[5]

Traditional Caribbean food isn't *South Beach Diet* food. The word "clean" is the main difference, as many of the same foods are consumed, but not the same quality. Clean Caribbean produce does much of the preliminary detoxification work with clean carbohydrates (roots, fruit, legumes, vegetables). Meanwhile, clean protein (meat, fish, dairy) and clean fats then provide the fuel for the detoxification engine. It is the traditional Caribbean foods and lifestyle that form the difference between the *South Beach Diet* and the Carefree system.

The best filtering process starts with eating clean, carefully selected food. Toxins that you don't ingest won't disrupt. Drink water that is purified so that you don't take in the toxins in modern water supply. Avoid hormonal problems by eating produce that doesn't have chemical buildup of pesticides or of heavily chemical-fertilized farming. Stop eating commercial meat and dairy so you won't suffer the nightmare of years of buildup of chemically doctored protein. Start eating seafood that the EWG ranks as clean.

Break away from grains, soy, commercial white potatoes, pasta, and other starches that transport man-made chemical toxins into the body that later must be fought with to get them to leave. Stop eating modern wheat products made from commercial stunt wheat, especially bread with its long list of chemical emulsifiers, additives, and preservatives.

No more seed oil "low-fat" processed foods so guilty of transporting trans fats into the body. Refuse to be tricked by multi-billion dollar food industry "healthy" fats made from vegetable oil, canola oil, safflower oil, and crushed seed oil.

Punched in the gut

Your gut is the front line battle zone of your health; the battle is won or lost there. Multiple clinical studies confirm that weightloss is directly an issue of the quality of what goes on in the gut, not exercise.[6,7,8] Weightloss, more specifically reduction of body fat, is interrupted by gastro-intestinal disorders. The GI lining is the mechanism that the body uses to manufacture roughly half of your neurotransmitters. The gut sends messengers to the brain where they are met by hormone receptors, leading to work orders for fat burning or fat retention.

Your goal should be to increase the microflora in the gut. This will raise the levels of glutathione, the primary human antioxidant. Glutathione is the body's sensation of good health, the anti-lethargy enzyme. Without active GI bacteria you'll produce insufficient neurotransmitters. This will lead to higher stress levels, low energy, low mood, low "spark" for exercise, then low "spark" for eating well. Indirectly this is one way that the lack of active GI bacteria leads to weight gain.

However, it's much more than providing energy or simply feeling better that so much attention should be directed to gut health. Research shows the toxic effect of herbicides on microbes in the soil.[9] Similar studies show the same problem: synthetic chemical compounds used in commercial agriculture kill off vast quantities of beneficial microflora in the soil. The soil is the starting point of gut microflora because crops absorb these organisms during growth. We eat the crops and the microbes move into our gut to join the ongoing battle for gut health. When modern industrial chemicals and antibiotics kill off microbiotica in the soil and then the food, the resulting gut dysfunction is weight gain.[10]

Chlorpyrifos is the most commonly used pesticide in the world. It's found in abundance on most commercial fruit and vegetables, including oranges, apples, tomatoes, and others. Although government agencies state that it is generally regarded as safe (GRAS) in produce consumption, it is death for microflora. You'll read that there is no proof that chlorpyrifos or other chemical farming agents kill people unless taking it in ridiculous quantities. This is true. But what is missing in the "safe" argument is what these fertilizers and pesticides do to vital microflora in the ground and so important in the gut. Once again, misinformation causes weight gain.

Microbiotica and weight control

It's sad that the "beer belly" images and the "pear shape" images are so woefully misunderstood. Right beneath the huge layer of fat is the GI tract, the reason for all that fat on the outside. We become obsessed with the outside, even seek liposuction to take it away, or maybe sit-ups to change the fat into six-pack abs. People tormented by their fat belly even get a cast put on around their waist to their chest in the faint hope removing the flab, a sign from the heavens that they have lost all sense of reason. How difficult can it be to re-think the problem? It's inside where the gut microflora resides that holds the key to all that fat on the outside.

Studies clearly show the direct connection between healthful gut microflora and maintaining optimal weight. One research team discovered that metabolic syndrome (abnormalities of the metabolic process related to obesity) increases inversely with the decrease in gut microbiotica.[11] A little time researching this theme will turn up dozens of peer reviewed studies pointing to the same thing: lack of gut microbiotica leads to problems of gaining weight.[12,13,14]

There is no connection between calorie counting, measuring carbohydrate grams, cutting out saturated fats, or yet another exercise program that will do anything to improve healthy microflora. What is overlooked in conventional wisdom is that the effort to maintain healthy gut microflora has a direct connection with your personal weightloss. Almost every conversation about weightloss will discuss calories, carbohydrates, and fats. Almost none of the conversations will discuss microflora – the real target you should be aiming at. As people debate the newest diet, "healthful" strawberries are passed around the table to munch on. Not one word will be spoken of the extremely high pesticide load on strawberries, even when washed with organic cleanser, and this toxin will enter the gut where it will attack microflora.

Furthermore, microflora health and its relationship to weightloss has a great deal to do with the diversity or variety of microbes in the gut. The greater diversity in the foods you eat the greater diversity in gut microbes you'll have. The greater diversity in gut microbes will provide optimal detoxing and weightloss capability.

It is by our choice in the foods we eat that we can protect or harm gut microbes. The high antibiotic content of commercial meat and dairy each have a devastating effect on gut microbes.[15] Processed foods, so laden with sugar and refined carbohydrates disrupt the function of gut microbes. Industrial seed oils (canola oil, safflower seed oil, corn oil, vegetable oil) have been found to have a toxic effect on healthy flora. Modern stunt wheat and especially the quantity of synthetic additives in commercial bread reduce beneficial microbes.

Finding salvation in the produce section

Good news, there is light in all of this toxic darkness. You can manipulate gut flora to your advantage. There are simple, every-day foods that build gut microbes and aid in weightloss efforts. Most of these are part of the traditional Caribbean diet and easily available at grocery stores. It is ordinary, cheap, every-day foods that should be your GI health instrument, not yet another magic powder from our multi-billion dollar food industry. Make sure you don't get suckered into taking another pill to fix your microflora problems, as thousands of years of standard Caribbean foods worked fine before the invention of pills.

Cruciferous vegetables are a corner piece to solving the puzzle of how to lose weight and help your gut microflora at the same time. Broccoli, cabbage, kale, and cauliflower are to be enjoyed several times per week. They have sulfur-containing glucosinolates that get broken down by microbes to reduce inflammation. Blueberries are another important source of GI health as they are rich in antioxidants with vitamin K compounds which diversify gut microbiotica. These berries are interwoven with Caribbean culture, grown throughout the region, and today Mexico is the world's top producer. Be very careful to only buy organic because berries are notoriously high in pesticides.

Yogurt is a great food for maintaining gut microflora but be careful with the quality. Standard grocery store yogurt with high sugar, preservatives, antibiotics and hormones would be a real bad choice. The source must be organic or grass fed, otherwise you get the joy of consuming the toxins which go into the animal feed, then more toxins into the milk production. Be sure to get full fat plain Greek yogurt to maximize the protein and probiotics. Is yogurt a traditional Caribbean food? No. But it doesn't matter because you'll use it as a topping on a meat dish or "ice cream" to have with fresh fruit. Life is good.

One of the easiest, cheapest, and most enjoyable ways to help your gut flora is through the consumption of resistant starch. Eaten in moderation, you'll lose weight without ever being hungry by feasting on green bananas (*plantains*), yuca (*cassabe*), sweet potato (*batata*), and pumpkin (*calabaza*).

The difficult part is accepting the change to these strange looking foods, to stop over-thinking it and just enjoy the flavorful meals. Obviously, adopting the Carefree Caribbean attitude makes all of this easy.

Plantains, sweet potatoes, yuca, and pumpkins are resistant starches that, when eaten, pass through the upper digestive tract thus stimulating good bacteria growth in the colon. These resistant starches increase fermentation and the production of short-chain fatty acids such as butyrate. These acids lower the pH for the bowel, making it less hospitable for bad bacteria. Butyrate is the preferred fuel of the cells that line the colon. Delicious Caribbean meals so abundant in resistant starches are perfect for stimulating gut bacteria growth.

Yet another food that is a rich source of health for your gut is fermented fiber, highly beneficial for cultivating gut microbiotica. The most common fermented fiber foods are sauerkraut or beet kimchi found in grocery stores. The popular Latin version of this is *curtido*. This is the spicy Central American fermented cabbage that ranges from moderately hot to the forest fire version. You can make your own or order this online (see Chapter 10).

Seafood toxins, a Caribbean tragedy

Seafood is instrumental to winning the battle of weightloss. This is a protein with unique omega-3 fatty acids that are reason alone to have seafood a couple of times per week. Its research-based effect on boosting brainpower should tell you to make certain it is part of your weekly diet. Then there are the natural sources of bioavailable minerals and micronutrients, not to mention the way seafood is interwoven with Caribbean culture. It is critical that you regularly eat seafood and regularly enjoy the process.

However, seafood toxins are so widespread that it has become a distressing part of the Carefree Caribbean Weightloss system. The West Indies developed as a seafood-based culture with a large fishing industry and diet that thrived on harvesting the Caribbean Sea. The clear blue seas provided a bounty of fresh seafood for human life since the first Mesoamerican settlers arrived more than 100 generations ago. Small fishing boats have always been part of the grand Caribbean culture; there are many songs about them. Ernest Hemingway's *Old Man and the Sea* pays homage to fishing the Caribbean waters off the coast of Cuba.

Industrial pollution has ruined the healthfulness of most Caribbean seafood, and seafood plays an essential part in the Carefree Caribbean Weightloss system. Very little of the enormous variety of seafood escapes the toxic effect, polluting King mackerel, Atlantic salmon, halibut, tuna, swordfish, shark, roughy, shrimp, and many others – each rated as dangerous by the EWG.[16]

Since you can't safely eat mercury contaminated fish from the Caribbean, you'll need to carefully shop for seafood with the lowest toxic rating. Although Atlantic salmon carries a dangerous rating, there is a salmon that carries an excellent rating. If the label states, "Wild Alaskan Salmon" this is a trademarked term that guarantees that the salmon will come from pristine northern waters, will not have been farm raised, and will therefore have very low levels of toxin. With Wild Alaskan Salmon, you can enjoy traditional Caribbean flavor and get the excellent nutrients and high amounts of omega-3 fatty acids into your diet. Best of all, Wild Alaskan Salmon is available in your nearby grocery store.

You can and should enjoy certain Caribbean shellfish and certain other seafood. Regularly make traditional Caribbean *ceviche*, that shellfish dish that is "cooked" in lime juice. It comes from seafood well down the food chain; oysters, octopus, squid, muscles and non-farm raised shrimp.

Another traditional Caribbean favorite is Island *paella*, that amazing saffron seasoned dish of oysters, octopus, squid, muscles and non-farm raised shrimp cooked with rice and vegetables. If you thaw a bag of frozen shellfish, it can be sautéed with garlic, olive oil, and spices in five minutes into fabulous *mariscos al ajillo*. The EWG also gives a thumbs up to enjoy lake trout, mackerel, sardines, anchovies, haddock, herring and pollock.

The criminal element is mercury. Worldwide coal fired electric plants with their enormous smokestacks send the soot to float hundreds of miles offshore. This soot is largely made up of the element mercury. The rains bring the mercury-soot into the seas where it is converted into highly toxic methylmercury that is absorbed by algae. Krill then eat the algae, larger fish eat the krill, and on up the food chain where the sharks eat at the top.

When humans eat mercury contaminated seafood, it binds with sulfur to disrupt protein metabolism causing a dietary domino effect. The mercury and sulfur then bind with iodine causing thyroid disruption, preventing the conversion of T4 into T3 hormone, with the result being weight gain.

In terms of its effect on the endocrine system, mercury damages cells in the pancreas that produce insulin, critical for the body's ability to metabolize sugar. Next, mercury causes mutations in the microbiome killing off good bacteria, critically effecting weight maintenance. Mercury is known to bioaccumulate in humans, where it can build up and effect the nervous system for a lifetime. And it's getting worse, as researchers have found that the problems of mercury exposure is growing much more rapidly than previously thought.[17]

Most people live in denial, refusing to believe the dire scientific warnings about toxins in seafood. You'll read that the entire mercury crisis is a fabrication of environmental crazies. In the face of multiple peer reviewed studies clearly showing the toxicity in seafood, people will tell you it's safe to eat all the fish you want, no matter what the mercury level is. (Aw shucks, a little mercury ain't gonna hurt.) However, with ample mercury-safe seafood readily available at your grocery store, it's a mystery why anyone would avoid eating seafood or agree to eat mercury loaded seafood.

Chemical sludge

Human toxic buildup was quite different in the past. Throughout history, food and water-borne toxins have killed populations at will, dysentery indiscriminately killed infants and adults, and water-borne cholera epidemics repeatedly wiped out thousands at a time. Starting in 1200 BC, Caribbean Islanders suffered terribly as flooding from hurricanes contaminated clean water repeatedly causing death and destruction.

But the last half century has brought in a separate misery – chemical toxins produced in industrial laboratories. Many of the pathogens that killed humanity in the past have been held under control by modern chemical additives.

There is a negative side to this. Today humans show the ill effects of this chemical overuse as it is applied to control bacteria in the environment. According to a report issued by the FDA, the governing agencies who watch over our national food and water supply currently allow over 3,000 synthetic chemicals to be consumed by humans.[18] It is only now that we experience the effects of these new chemicals, as though discovering the side effects of strong medicine.

Contaminated water has forever been one of the great killers of civilization. Although nowhere near as deadly, it is a danger to mankind today as it was in the past. What weapon was used by the Spanish *conquistadors* to wipe out 20 million natives? Contaminated water killed millions while guns killed hundreds. Native Americans had no immunity defense against the common cold, flu, and infectious diseases of the *conquistadors*. A common cold for a Spanish soldier was passed by water to defenseless natives, and death was almost certain. One fever-ravaged native could infect thousands of fellow natives simply by washing in a common river. As a biological counter attack, the natives offered sexually transmitted diseases, as the Spanish raped and pillaged, they had no immunity from the forms of syphilis in the Americas.

The western world today has largely eradicated most water-borne disease. In its place we now must slowly suffer from the effects of chemicals permitted in drinking water. Lead, mercury, cadmium, drug residue, pesticides, jet fuel leakage, and petroleum based fertilizers join a host of other toxins that go into the water and don't come out. Researchers have repeatedly stated that there is no safe dosage of lead for humans. Even if by some miracle your tap water was pure when it arrived at your nice new house, studies show that lead toxins from the plumbing fixtures enter drinking water.

Water toxins are a major concern for those seeking to lose weight, as contaminants become hormonal disruptors and a source of weight gain. The best cure is to install a good quality purified water apparatus to your tap, not plastic bottled water that seeps toxins from the plastic to the water.

From the chemical lab to livestock feed, then to us

"Why should we tolerate a diet of weak poisons."
  ~ Rachel Carson

Our modern industrial meat supply is very effective at chemically fighting bacteria. Consider that 25.8 billion pounds of commercial beef is served to Americans each year and results in very few cases of botulism or e-coli poisonings; we should feel safe. Adding poultry and pork, the number tops 50 billion pounds of meat in our national diet.

However the way meat is made safe from disease is hardly safe. Modern industrial meat mostly comes from confined animal feeding operations (CAFOs) that make the process economically efficient. Being incredibly cramped with as many as a million birds under one roof, with shoulder to shoulder cattle literally living in their own excrement, costly animal disease is rampant.

CAFO livestock is therefore fed or injected with antibiotics to avoid disease and with hormones to make the animals grow to the most profitable huge size. They are fed corn and soy specifically designed to rapidly fatten them up for market. To insure that this massive amount of meat makes it safely to market, they are given mind boggling quantities of antibiotics to stay alive. More than 80% of all antibiotics sold in the United States are used for livestock production.[19]

For example, just in North Carolina, the quantity of antibiotics used in livestock feed has been estimated to exceed all US antibiotic use in human medicine. Conventional wisdom responds that it is needed and won't hurt us. However, the World Health Organization (WHO) disagrees. Studies have found that European bans on antibiotic use for livestock and poultry production hasn't had any negative effect on animal health.[20] It's the financial health of the chemical producers and providers who get hurt by banning chemicals in the meat supply.

Due to our refusal to end antibiotic treatment of animals, meat from the US is banned in many countries. As the FDA reported, sales of antibiotics to be fed to pigs, chicken, cattle and seafood rose 20% between the years 2009 and 2013. Recently the FDA admitted that 32.6 million pounds of antibiotics were either fed or injected into US commercial meat, and most of the antibiotics were given in frequent low doses which results in faster growth in CAFO pens.[21]

All of the antibiotics and growth hormones routinely given to CAFO animals serve to make them incredibly fat. This is what we eat when we order beef, pork, chicken, turkey or farm raised seafood at a restaurant. Restaurants and grocery stores sell this meat with the perfectly legal claim of "100% natural" meat.

Once again, misinformation plagues us as dietitians or personal trainers encourage cutting off the fat of this meat, to avoid frying it to cut back on fats, but to eat the meat anyway. They are right when they say that hormones and antibiotics in livestock won't cause cancer or heart disease. However, not once will the discussion be about CAFO meat harming microflora. This misinformation talks on and on about calories, fats and carbohydrates, and drowns out discussion about how commercial meat leads to hormonal dysfunction and ultimately to weight gain.[22]

Antibiotics disrupt gut microflora, killing off bacteria and changing the balance of flora species in the intestines. Studies have found that babies who received antibiotics in the first six months of life, just when their microbiome was evolving, became fatter.[23] There is a growing belief in the scientific community that chronic repeated low-dose exposure to antibiotics significantly contributes to weight gain, and we get that exposure in standard restaurant or grocery store meat.

According to research published in the *Proceedings of the National Academy of Sciences*, commercial pigs have the highest antibiotics in their meat, followed by chicken, then beef. Researchers note that farm raised salmon, shrimp, tilapia and other fish have at least five different antibiotics in their meat.[24] The water around or downstream from animal CAFO feeding farms have extremely high levels of antibiotics.

One major problem with CAFO meat is the fact that it has almost entirely made up of omega-6 fatty acids. This causes a chronic imbalance in fatty acids. With a couple of hours of study you can easily find a dozen peer reviewed studies showing that the overconsumption of omega-6 fats leads to weight gain.[25] Your diet must place high emphasis on limiting omega-6 fatty acids and focusing on consuming more omega-3 to have any chance of maintaining a balance.[26] This a compelling reason avoid CAFO meat and instead eat range free livestock, poultry, eggs and wild caught Alaska salmon, all of which feature omega-3 fatty acids.

What's not listed on the label

We proudly consume meat without the slightest notion what's in it. 100% lean USDA inspected ground beef can cause you to gain weight, and it has nothing to do with saturated fat or red meat. High quantities of industrial toxins include petroleum based fertilizer or pesticides are used to grow the cattle feed. In minute amounts, these chemicals become part of the 100% beef paddy.[27, 28] Commercial ground beef has a huge list of chemical additives including:

Sodium benzoate, butylated hydroxyanisole, butylated hydroxy toluene, dichlorobenzene, trichloroethane, trimethylbenzene, tetrachloroethylene, dyphnyl 2-ethylhexyl phosphate, ethyl benzene, octachlor epoxide, toluene, chlorpyrifos, diazinon, iprodione, propyl benzene, and other synthetic chemicals.

Processed meats, pepperoni, beef jerky, and hot dogs are brimming with additives including sodium nitrate, sodium acid pyrophosphate, and glucona delta lactone. The favorite spices in hot dogs are often spiked with monosodium glutamate, a neurotoxin that is linked to weight gain and brain damage. The USDA states that all hot dogs are tested and well below the maximum level for additives established.[29] Then the food industry plays a cruel trick of offering CAFO low-fat chicken or turkey meat to replace evil red meat hot dogs as a way to attract health conscious buyers. All this meat is safe, we are told.

However, in a recent symposium of 22 toxicologists from ten countries it was found that the people who regularly consume processed meat are at carcinogenic risk much greater than previously thought.[30] The main culprit is sodium nitrite, added to fix the color of the meat from a grayish hue to fresh looking pink. Sodium nitrite also helps keep hot dogs and other processed meats on shelves for weeks, and more weeks at home in the refrigerator. In the early 1970's, the USDA tried to ban sodium nitrite but was forced to stop their efforts because of intense political influence from the meat industry. Half a century later we are swimming in sodium nitrate.

Eat chicken breasts, we are told. Nobody asks what kind of chicken. The story begins with what the bird puts in its stomach and the soil that the chicken feed comes from. US chicken feed starts off with 170 million acres devoted to growing corn and soy. To grow corn and soy, the ground is first saturated with truckloads of petroleum/nitrogen based fertilizer. These fertilizers have caused human birth defects in crop growing regions, have caused field workers to prematurely die, and must be handled with hazardous chemical protective clothing.[31]

However, the USDA states that none of these truckloads of fertilizer wind up in the corn and soy crops. If the toxic chemicals aren't sucked into the plant, it's a mystery where it all goes. Reassuringly, we are told by the USDA that commercial grains are safe to eat.[32]

Crops for chicken feed are further treated with toxic pesticides to kill of weeds, fungi, insects and rodents. Chicken feed is then supplemented with dried blood and pulverized chicken carcasses to raise the protein levels and make chicks grow. Added to the feed is a substance called Roxarsone, which is arsenic to increase growth.[33] It is safe, we are told.

As the chick experiences spectacular growth, more toxins are added to the feed with high amounts of antibiotics and growth hormones. In weeks the chick grows so fat it can hardly walk, but instead lives in a room as large as an aircraft hangar wall-to-wall with rapidly growing chicks. Seven weeks after birth, five pound broiler chicks are slaughtered and shipped to market.

Dairy go round

You'll hear arguments on both sides of the debate about whether dairy is good for weightloss or not. Some arguments are about lactose intolerance and sweeteners added to cream. But the big debates are about fats. Cheese, butter, ice cream and yogurt get judged by fat content.

However, saturated fats of milk pose little problem with weightloss.[34] In fact, low-fat on a dairy label is sign that the content makes you fatter due to the additional sugars added to make up for the missing fat.

Conventional wisdom states that Dannon strawberry yogurt is good for you because it's just yogurt and strawberries. The label's list of ingredients won't inform you that the long list of additives in the yogurt and the strawberries are a serious weight gain trigger, but you're sure to see the calorie count. As you watch people proudly eating this yogurt with "fresh fruit" as they boast of their healthful diet, what you are seeing is people making themselves fat.

Commercial milk products have another health hazard. Milk comes from cows that live on a steroid diet leading to phenomenal growth but early death. The antibiotics, synthetic chemical feed, and toxins in drinking water all pass through the cow into the milk in tiny amounts that gradually build up in humans. Then there is the problem of rBGH.

In 1993, the FDA approved recombinant bovine growth hormone (rBGH), a synthetic hormone that spurs milk production when injected into dairy cows. The scientific community and consumer groups have been alarmed about it ever since, to no avail. Naturally, conventional wisdom states that since the government says milk has no problem with rBGH, it's safe.

This miracle drug originally from Monsanto Chemical stimulates up to 20% more milk production out of every cow. Monsanto pushed to get rBGH approved in the US despite strong opposition from scientists who warned of a health crisis if this hormone were to be approved.[35] Not only did the Food and Drug Administration approve it, the Environmental

Protection Agency continues to license it today. Soon after the approval of rBGH, the FDA ruled that rBGH dairy products did not have to have the hormone listed on the label. Today in your grocery store, by law, your milk or yogurt label won't include rBGH on the ingredients list but it will list fat content and calories.

The late Professor Samuel Epstein of the University of Illinois was the well-respected chairman of the Cancer Prevention Coalition. He made a compelling case for avoiding commercial products and their ever-present rBGH.[36] Epstein believed that natural milk is different from rBGH milk nutritionally, pharmacologically, immunologically, and hormonally. The major differences with rBGH milk include:

1. *Increased levels of thyroid hormone enzyme thyroxin-5'-monodeiodinase.*
2. *rBGH milk has imbalanced levels of insulin growth factor-1 (IGF-1).*
3. *Cows get injected with antibiotics and drugs to treat mastitis and other rBGH-induced diseases.*
4. *This milk has an increased concentration of omega-6 over omega-3 fatty acids.*

This frightening rBGH hormone additive is banned throughout Europe, Canada, Japan, and most of the industrialized world. Although there are no known direct links between rBGH treated milk and obesity or weight gain, there are strong indicators that it plays a "building block" role.[37] When combined with a multitude of toxins in the standard American diet, rBGH milk fuels other directly linked obesity toxins. Especially problematic is that rBGH is a building block for IGF-1. For twenty years studies have consistently shown that there is a direct link between an excess of IGF-1 and obesity.[38] This is in the commercial milk, cream, ice cream, cheese, and yogurt we consume. It is safe, we are told.

Produce from hell, produce form heaven

"By their very nature, most pesticides create some risk of harm to humans, animals, or the environment because they are designed to kill or otherwise adversely affect living organisms."

~ US Environmental Protection Agency

Lettuce, spinach, and kale are sponges for chemical fertilizers and pesticides. These delicate plants are heavily dosed with herbicides, fungicides, insecticides, along with dozens of toxins in fertilization, soil preparation, and preservation. More so than thick skinned vegetable cousins, the typical leafy greens of a salad are easy targets for sucking up chemical toxins from the ground and absorbing more toxic pesticides sprayed from the air. Misinformation has us faithfully eating our salad without knowing what was is actually inside. To add insult to it, we are talked into buying a special wash to remove residue from the outside of the leaves somehow forgetting that the inside has even more toxins.

Commercial tomatoes are almost as bad. After petroleum based fertilizer prepared the soil, there is a frightening list of chemicals sprayed over the ground as pesticides to protect the tomato crop. These pesticides for tomatoes literally form an independent industry. Sulphur is the most commonly used. Other widely used pesticides are chlorpyrifos, metam potassium, 1.3-dichloropropene, and sodium hypo-chlorite. In 2005, California tomato fields used 1,055,085 gross pounds of pesticides, made up of 49 separate chemical compounds. By 2015 that amount increased by 4%, with a large portion flowing into streams and rivers, eventually making their way to drinking water and oceans.[39]

The Environmental Working Group ranks the pesticide level of most produce eaten today. Based on the analysis of 28,000 samples, their ranking of clean to unclean means that several important vegetables should be only be purchased as organic. The EWG rates the worst pesticide-loaded vegetables to be:

Bell peppers (all colors)	Celery
Cucumbers	Green beans, string beans
Hot peppers	Kale
Russet potatoes	Spinach
Snap peas	Tomatoes
Winter squash	

The EWG also ranks fruit as clean to unclean. The worst pesticide-loaded fruit should only come from organic sources. The EWG rates the worst pesticide-loaded fruit to be:

Apples   Cherries
Grapes   Peaches
Pears   Nectarines
Strawberries (worst ranking of all produce)

Artificial additives

Nearly a century ago a scientist in Germany accidentally mixed several chemicals together and found that the lab smelled like grapes. This discovery of methyl anthranilate was the first widespread synthetic flavor. Later, methyl anthranilate became famous when it became the basic grape flavor of Kool-Aid. Soft drinks today continue to use the highest amount of methyl anthranilate flavor additives, although it is also heavily used in candy and gum.

American buyers seem to be addicted to artificial flavors. Moving down the grocery store isle, you can note that the label on the bottle says, "natural and artificial flavors." This is the legal term for adding a small amount of industrial chemical toxins to food. What's in that stuff you're eating? The healthy yogurt with banana flavor comes from an ester called isoamyl acetate. When you have a health bar with almond flavor, you're eating benzaldehyde, often made of the ester called octyl acetate. This chemical has been repeatedly shown to cause central nervous system convulsions and depression.[40]

Anything with artificial vanilla flavor has vanillin, chemically known as 4-hydroxy-3methoxy-benzaldehyde. This compound is surprisingly added to "healthy" cranberry raisinets among other products. It is made from the waste products of paper mills mixed with petroleum. When you buy something with pear flavor, you're buying amyl acetate. This chemical compound causes nervous system depression, headaches, and fatigue.[41]

But it is cinnamon that is the most difficult to understand. Artificial cinnamon flavor is made from synthetic cinnamyl formate, or formic acid. Compare that to real cinnamon (mostly from Ceylon) which is the bark of the cinnamomum verum tree, ground to a powder. This spice has been used for centuries as an herb for health and flavor. British traders brought it to the Caribbean centuries ago where today it is an integral part of the West Indies diet, including its use in Jamaican jerk seasoning. While artificial cinnamon comes from a chemical factory, true cinnamon is a tremendous aid to health and weightloss. And we buy the artificial one.

Why use synthetic lab concoctions when the natural plant is easy to buy, easy to use, tastes better, and aids in health? The answer is the power of marketing misinformation.

HFCS nightmare

Corn is a major player in our modern society and economy. It feeds us, fuels our cars, is transformed into carboard boxes and even gets fabricated into toilets. And it is made into modern sugar.

In the 1970's the world was introduced to the first mass-scale industrial sweetener, high fructose corn syrup (HFCS). This is the story of corn's path from thousands of years of healthful corn grown to feed Latin America to a high-tech process right out of a science fiction movie.

HFCS is an ultra-sweet syrup made for pennies compared to the problematic and more expensive sugar. Treated with an enzyme that converts glucose to fructose, HFCS results in a product that tastes many times sweeter than sugar. It also preserves, saving even more money for food producers. Within its first few years, HFCS production exploded.

To manufacture HFCS, first you need vast quantities of field corn, that corn so different from the corn on the cob we all enjoy. The corn is milled to make corn starch, a carbohydrate consisting of long chains of glucose. The corn starch is diluted, then enzymes are added to break down the glucose into shorter chains of glucose. More enzymes are added to reduce the glucose to molecules. The end syrup is a financial miracle for farmers.

Over 50% of adults drink up to six sugary beverages weekly, and these are the main source of dietary HFCS. About 33% of adults drink one HFCS beverage every day. In that there was a 1,000% HFCS consumption increase between 1970 and 1990, clearly this super sweet syrup has an addictive hold on people. By 2009, American adult consumption of HFCS was 35.7 pounds, as proudly reported by the Illinois Farm Bureau.

It's hard to get people to eat healthful fresh fruit that isn't sweet enough when packaged fruit swimming in HFCS tastes much sweeter. HFCS is in foods you would never expect; in almost every beverage in the store, in almost every sauce or dressing, peanut butter, soups, ice cream, ketchup, pickles and relish, plus an endless quantity of other products. Soft drinks are sweetened with HFCS, but also "pure" apple juice, canned corn, processed meats, and another estimated 4,000 food products.

To keep from getting fat, conventional wisdom says to eat low-fat turkey breast. However, HFCS is added to this along with a long list of synthetic chemicals found in processed turkey slices and other processed meat.

It is no coincidence that in the years since the introduction of HFCS, we have experienced our current obesity epidemic. Although it would be incorrect to say HFCS is the root cause of obesity, it clearly plays an important part. Many scientists believe HFCS to be addictive and a major contributor to the obesity epidemic.[42] Coupled with the prevalence of HFCS in vast quantities of products, researchers fear that this leads to a national craving for everything to taste sweet. Worst of all, HFCS has institutionalized sweetness; a generation of addicts who demand sweetness and are unfamiliar with the lack of sweetness.

Unpronounceable chemicals we swallow

The website for American International Chemical Corporation lists fifteen separate chemicals sold to meat processors to "improve yield, enhance water, fat and protein binding, improve manufacturability, and enhance the shelf life requirements of both cooked and uncooked processed meat products." These include:

Erythorbic acid, fumaric acid, lucono-delta lactone, malic acid, pirosil (silicon dioxide), potassium lactate, potassium nitrate, potassium sorbate, sodium benzoate, sodium carboxmethylcellulose (CMC), sodium diacetate, sodium erythorbate, sodium nitrate, sorbic acid, tricalcium phosphate.

We blindly snack on processed food loaded with synthetic chemical compounds to enjoy "food" that was built to last on the shelves for months. We pay extra for "health foods" but fail to look at the list of chemical additives and fail to look up what those additives do to humans. Then we read in respected international scientific journals, yet again, that synthetic chemicals lead to weight gain, and then…nothing happens. Instead we turn to soothsayers who tell us that it's calories, excess fat, and not enough exercise. And the chemical industry churns out more.

And we swallow it, no questions asked

"The real question is what is happening at low doses as opposed to what is happening at high doses."
~ Dr. Linda Birnbaum, President, Society of Toxicology

Industrially processed food is another term for artificial additives. Processed foods are almost always have artificial color, artificial texture, artificial flavor, and a long list of preservatives. There are additives for "mouth feel", additives "for better flavor", additives "to promote color retention", and a list of other compelling reasons why this or that synthetic chemical was added.

On average, every man, woman, and child ingests 3.5 pounds of chemical additives per year, consumed a drop at a time.[43] Not one dose of this is lethal. You won't go blind form a day's ingestion and you'll never need to race to the hospital emergency room because of your daily chemical dose. The FDA considers all additives to be safe.

Do we need foods to have artificial bright color for our health? In American foods, we use over 3,000 tons of artificial color each year. It is highly concentrated so that a few droplets of coloring are all that is needed to color a large quantity of food. Packaged meat and energy bars sell better when brightly colored, but fresh oranges also sell better when chemically treated with highly toxic Red Dye #40 to improve color (and sales) while breakfast cereals look more attractive and sell better with the widespread use of Yellow Dye #5. Yellow dye is widely used in cheeses, pickles, canned fruits, sauces, and especially chips. Blue Dye #1 is popular in energy drinks and candy. It's all safe, we are told.

A massive study of 12,000 people by the National Academy of Sciences found that we ingest as much as 200 milligrams of food dyes per day.[44] Although no one will be killed by this, the cumulative effect is the danger. When a meal consists of tiny droplets of food dye blended with a tiny dose of emulsifier in bakery goods and a tiny bit of potassium sorbate for flavoring and a tiny bit of texturizer and a tiny bit of preservative and a tiny bit of sodium nitrate – we have a serious chemical additive problem. However, the government agencies who are paid to protect us measure one chemical only, failing to address the cumulative effect. So we are stuck with government assessments of safety based upon one chemical, not on one total day of collective chemical consumption.

For two decades we have known of the health hazards form chemical food additives. The World Health Organization began issuing warnings in 1999 after viewing the effects of dietary industrial toxins. They found that the typical levels consumed to be an international health hazard and issued wide-spread warnings. Every year the WHO has repeatedly issued warnings and impact statements from their offices in Switzerland.

In the United States, the results have been precisely zero. The last decade has seen a vast increase in synthetic chemicals into our food supply. While WHO warns of the dangers, we are told by manufacturers, government watchdogs, doctors, dietitians, and health specialists that everything is safe. Just watch your calories, eat low fat food, and exercise more.

Save yourself by going to the grocery store, buy clean food, bring it home to cook it with flourish, then ceremoniously dine on your creation. And yes, be sure to sip some sangria and nibble on dark chocolate as you nod to the food industry. They may fool most people but they can't fool all.

Seven

ENDOCRINE DISRUPTING CHEMICALS

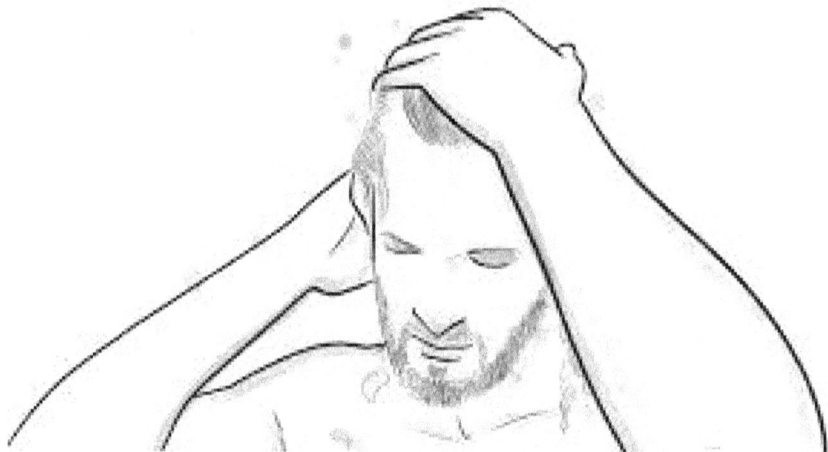

"My hypothesis is that chemicals are the basis behind the global health epidemic, because at the levels of chemicals we are being exposed to, they're poisoning our weight control systems, which is damaging our ability to lose weight and make us fatter."
~ Paula Baille-Hamilton, MD

After Dr. Ballie-Hamilton gave birth to her second child, she gained twenty pounds and had no success at losing weight. Her standard medical training told her that the problem was that she took in too many calories and didn't burn them off. But then her scientific mind didn't buy in to that assumption.

The more she studied, the more she found other researches had come to the same conclusion that calorie counting is a dead end. These researchers found that there are thousands of synthetic chemicals in our diet, kitchen, laundry room and home environment that team up to disrupt hormones leading to weight gain. Over the last decade, researchers have found evidence that these compounds add body weight and hold on to it despite the calories consumed or calories expended.

The culprit is the way various man-made chemicals force naturally occurring hormones to fail. Hormones that are supposed to help in weightloss become chemically altered to not function or function in the wrong way. The intricate wiring of the endocrine system with its checks and balances, just stops working right. It works but not the way it could.

To avoid these chemically altered hormones begins with a better understanding. In a sea of synthetic chemicals, we are all cast adrift unless we study what is going wrong and what to do to make things work right. In order to take control of your health and weightloss, much of your effort will similarly need to turn your back on conventional wisdom and look instead to your endocrine system. In this effort, there is another dose of science needed.

Without getting bogged down into biochemistry, at least get familiar with the danger zones. The science shouldn't get in your way or scare you off from the information that will help you live better and a lot thinner. Just breeze through the biochemistry so as to familiarize yourself with the essentials.

Synthetic chemicals that disrupt or copy hormones cause serious problems in health and especially in causing weight gain. They are commonly referred to as endocrine disruptors (EDs) or endocrine disrupting chemicals (EDCs). These toxic chemicals directly lead to a wide range of damage to the endocrine system, and if left unchecked, can lead to permanent damage.

EDs reduce production of certain hormones.
EDs increase production of others.
EDs turn one hormone into another.
EDs confuse the body with hormone imposters.
EDs interfere with signaling hormones.
EDs command cells to die prematurely.
EDs bind to hormones.
EDs accumulate in organs that produce hormones.
EDs chronically interrupt digestion of nutrients.

EDs have a terrible effect on sex hormones. Changes in sex hormones are clinically known to cause weight gain, and cellular damage from pesticides damage sex hormones.[1, 2] We don't even have to consume them as pesticides on food or drink them from contaminated water to have them cause weight gain. Labor saving household products such as non-stick lining on pans or plastic lining to protect food in the refrigerator disrupt sex hormones and essentially lock fat to the body.

Obesogens: an unseen invasion

"One of the most pernicious ramifications of obesogens is that their effects can be passed on to future generations. That's right: the effects of obesogen exposure can be heritable."
~ Dr. Bruce Blumberg, University of California Irvine

The science of EDs was given a jump start in 2006 by the work of Dr. Bruce Blumberg, an eminent researcher from the University of California Irvine. His team of researchers found that some fish in the nearby harbor were fat while others of the same species were normal.

The fish lived near each other and had the same diet, but the fat ones were in regular contact with small boats, feeding right next to them. The chemicals leeching from the paint on the boats was affecting the fat fish while their cousins stayed lean. This was the genesis of Blumberg's discovery of obesogens, or synthetic chemicals that cause obesity. Obesogens are the worst of the worst endocrine disruptors.

Most humans have not been poisoned to the point of no return, and with a drastic change can avoid being like Blumberg's fish. For Blumberg's fish, those that did not have direct contact with the paint did not yet get obese. The normal fish could easily have a fish family reunion under the ED contaminated boat with obesity as a result. The fish metaphor is made to be a stern warning. Avoid dangerous chemicals that surround you or pay the consequences.

Dr. Blumberg's latest book, *The Obesogen Effect: Why We Eat Less and Exercise More but Still Struggle to Lose Weight* shows how his internationally acclaimed hormone research has led to a reversal in the understanding of weightloss. Gone are the days of seeing weight gain or loss being a balance of calories in and calories out. Now is the time to see the worst EDs guilty of storing fat and regulating the metabolism.

Basically, the toxic chemical invasion of the last century has exhausted the primary human detoxification mechanism, the liver. Overwhelmed by demands placed upon it, the liver functions at a small percentage of its capability. In this weakened state, insulin resistance takes hold in a downward spiral to obesity. However, the human body is remarkably resilient. Over time with changes in lifestyle and diet, the liver can bounce back to much better and even to an optimal detoxification potential. That is, if it is given the chance to break free from the chemical onslaught now. In effect, the liver must be given some time to rest and recover.

Recently the International Endocrine Society task force issued a statement on EDs, pointing out that the health effects of endocrine disrupting chemicals are so severe that everyone needs to take proactive steps to avoid them.[3] Due to the pervasive nature of EDs, well-advertised weightloss products will do nothing to change the fat producing EDs in your life until you remove them.

When allowed to, EDs interfere with or disrupt normal hormone function. This leads to a wide range of human health disasters including cancerous tumors, birth defects, learning disabilities, anatomical deformities, developmental disorder, and obesity. EDs are quite stable, thus they don't break down quickly. Since they can be added to foods and tend to stabilize the product, many food manufacturers include them in products as a form of preservative.[4,5] The stability of ED's means they last for a very long time in water, soil, grocery store shelves, and in the human body.

Roadblock to weightloss

"Progress is impossible without change, and those who cannot change their minds cannot change anything."
    ~ George Bernard Shaw

Endocrine disruptors directly affect whether you gain weight or lose weight.[6] ED's promote obesity by altering metabolism, fat cell signaling, glucose uptake, increasing inflammation, and increasing appetite. Even very small amounts of EDs can have a major impact. For this reason, EDs are often measured in ppt (parts per trillion).

The Environmental Working Group lists the 12 most common EDs, of which 10 are in the food and water supply, and all are directly linked to weight gain.[7] While pesticides cause many health problems, one of the worst problems for people trying to lose weight is that these pesticides in our food supply are EDs mimicking estrogen. The result is similar to getting injected with estrogen, disrupting the body's ability to build lean muscle instead of promoting fat storage.

Nearly 1,000 EDs are listed on the Endocrine Disruption Exchange, with 18 documented as obesogens.[8] When EDs eventually become stored in fat cells, their volume becomes proportional to body fat volume. The more body fat, the more EDs have likely been stored. Because they also disrupt immune function, they tend to leave people weak with "lingering colds" and associated illness. With energy sapped it becomes a constant feeling of listlessness and lack of well-being.

Decreasing production of some hormones, increasing production of others, converting one hormone into another, imitating yet another hormone; EDs actively prevent loss of weight. They signal hormones to act the opposite of a normal healthy human; commonly ingested EDs actually signal healthy cells to die young. The most virulent EDs, obesogens, change metabolic function, alter fat storage, disrupt energy balance, and interfere with regulation of appetite.

A library of research confirms the direct connection between the enormous amount of pesticides in our food supply and resulting endocrine disruption. Researchers have found that pesticide overuse has a much more tragic effect on hormonal health than previously believed.[9] The consumption of industrially processed foods that are so laden with residue from pesticides and synthetic compounds will block your efforts to lose weight no matter what diet you are on or what workout you do.

We get these EDs from a variety of foods and even from household products. These products seem so harmless, so normal that it is easier to get people to avoid the EDs in foods than it is to get them to avoid household ED sources like shampoo and fragrances. People seem to believe that non-stick cookware, air-fresheners in the car, toilet cleansers, and deodorants couldn't possibly be so bad.

Bold faced lies

In the face evidence that EDs directly cause weight gain, the entire weightloss industry has pretty much buried its head in the sand. Many of the problems of losing weight in general and hormone disruption specifically come from having ample information that is simply ignored. Instead, we feast on misinformation. It happens with one mistaken nutritional idea leading to the next and the next and so on. Then when confronted with the misinformation, we step back to the safety zone of conventional wisdom. We have grown accustomed to the misinformation.

One of the worst moments of dietary misinformation happened in 1961. There the infamous Lipid Hypothesis of Dr. Ancel Keys made the cover of Time magazine, pointing a finger at saturated fats as the cause of heart disease. The media latched on and modern society went to war with saturated fats for 50 years.[10] The war on saturated fats still rages on, even though no evidence passes scientific muster that saturated fats cause people to get fat. Even today most of the practitioners in weightloss adhere to the evil saturated fat narrative.

The argument took a turn for the worse immediately after it was hatched. Since saturated fats were "obviously" bad, there was a gold rush for unsaturated fats such as margarine and the horrors of trans fats, perhaps the most dangerous food product every introduced to mankind. Trans fats are unsaturated fats, "partially hydrogenated vegetable oil" which offered longer shelf life and better stability of a vast array of foods. Today these fats are directly linked to heart disease, and today are increasingly banned from use in restaurants. But for half a century, mankind gobbled up trans fats in part because they were "good" unsaturated fats.

The next bit of misinformation was that soy could save us from the horrors of saturated fats because soy has only about 6% saturated fats and is brimming with protein. We then turned to massive industrial soy production as a solution, bringing soy milk, soy baby formula, and soy products to every home in the western world.

These soy products are a hormonal nightmare, leaving the ill effects of phytoestrogens as a by-product. Phytoestrogens are plant hormone copycats that hinder the function of our natural hormonal process. Specifically, soy is terrible for thyroid health, and thyroid health is essential to weightloss. Soy products come with multiple negative effects on mineral absorption, and it is the absence of sufficient calcium, magnesium, iron, and zinc that is directly linked to increased stress. It is the ED properties of genistein, the primary isoflavone in soy that is at the center of most research into the hormonal damage from soy.[11]

Of all the food products we consume, soy is the most genetically modified. To make matters worse, massive industrial soy production uses genetically modified soy, and the resulting GMO phytoestrogens are a major endocrine disruptor. They mimic estrogen and block receptor sites against normal estrogen – the result is often to lock abdominal fat to the body.[12] As a direct result of the modern fear of saturated fat, the soy industry has exploded in growth and influence on national food policy.

Perhaps the worst misinformation in regard to obesity and weightloss has come from the weightloss industry itself, in this case, calorie counting. Decades ago this calorie mania took the form of artificial sweeteners, as sugar was high in calories and therefore "bad" while artificial chemical lab sweeteners were therefore "good" because they had no calories. Rather than read the list of artificial sugar's unpronounceable chemicals, people were essentially told to shut up and just count the calories.

No one seemed to care what was in those artificial sweetener chemical compounds or the effect they would have on the human body. Because calories were considered evil and pretty much the same, packages of artificial sweetener were put on every table in every restaurant as a coffee sweetener.

With artificial sweeteners, mankind experienced a massive disruption of endocrine function, including epidemic thyroid dysfunction. Although research on a direct link between artificial sweeteners and endocrine damage doesn't exist, there is growing fear that low thyroid dysfunction may well be made worse by artificial sweeteners.

Low thyroid output is directly connected with increased body fat, and rather than fix mankind's new thyroid crisis, we were once again told to count calories and consume more "healthful" foods such as artificial sweeteners. Even today many "health" drinks have a generous portion of artificial sweeteners straight out of the chemical plant. The supposed magical Amazon acai berry, pro-biotic drinks, protein shakes, energy drinks, green superfood drinks, energy boost pink lemonade, Muscle Milk, and dozens of other popular "health" drinks each use artificial sweeteners. And sales are booming.

Glyphosate inside you

"Our gut bacteria contains the same metabolic pathway found in plants targeted and disrupted by RoundUp. Is it any wonder that leaky gut syndrome, IBD, colitis and other gastrointestinal diseases have spiked since the onset of RoundUp Ready GMO crops?"

~ Dr. Stephanie Seneff, Senior Research Scientist, MIT

The poster child for modern dietary misinformation is glyphosate, Monsanto's RoundUp. This is an endocrine disrupting obesogen that, with regular microscopic ingestion, will most certainly make you fat on the way to serious disease. An entire land mass of agricultural America is repeatedly sprayed with this fierce antibiotic to kill weeds in order for more crops to grow. We consume this extremely dangerous ED a droplet at a time in a variety of ways.

Scientific data about the health danger of glyphosate is consistently presented to government health agencies by some of the most esteemed scientists in the nation. After a study of glyphosate and other pesticides was conducted and published in *Endocrine Reviews*, one such research team stated, "Experimental data indicate that EDCs and hormones do not have NOELs [no observed adverse effect level] or threshold doses, and therefore no dose can ever be considered safe."[13]

Professor Stephanie Seneff of MIT has sounded the alarm about glyphosate for more than 10 years, has been published in the top scientific journals and regularly lectures on the health crisis created by glyphosate. Her argument is that the human endocrine system is permanently damaged by exposure to this widely used product, and despite the data to show its danger, it continues to be widely applied to our every-day foods.

Glyphosate causes a range of health problems, but especially obesity.[14] It is widely used on cattle feed, along with antibiotics, growth hormones, and many other toxic chemicals. By disrupting bacterial homeostasis in human enzymes, glyphosate severely disrupts serotonin production and delivery. Since serotonin is a signaling mechanism intertwined with ghrelin, the actions of both hormones are mutually disrupted by glyphosate.

According to multiple studies, glyphosate depletes the amino acids tyrosine, tryptophan, and phenylalanine, the results of which can contribute to obesity, depression, autism, inflammatory bowel disease, Alzheimer's and Parkinson's.[15] As a nation, we have taken the attitude that "it can't be that bad" and therefore allow glyphosate to harm us all.

Dr. Seneff states that glyphosate is arguably "…the most important factor in the development of multiple chronic diseases and conditions that have become prevalent in Westernized societies." After hounding government agencies, international lectures, research papers, and dozens of news interviews, the result of this warning is almost zero. There has been no reduction in glyphosate use.

If you want to find some glyphosate in your home, just open a jar of peanut butter, or open a frozen pizza, have a bowl of cereal, or eat any number of packages of processed food. Glyphosate is used extensively in wheat and soy production, so much that it has been found in Wheaties,

Trix, Cheerios, Quaker Oats, and Lucky Charms. The farmlands of grain that get drenched in glyphosate then pass it on to commercial grain-fed livestock, and then into our food supply. Glyphosate sprayed grain is found in commercially sold granola and crackers, so much so that more than 8,000 lawsuits have been filed against Monsanto, one of which resulted in a $289 million legal settlement.

This ED is unregulated in non-food applications; thus it is profusely used in cotton fields. It turns out that cotton and peanut crops are rotated in the same field for maximum yield, and the peanut crops then get a volatile load of glyphosate left over in the soil. Peanut butter is a major source of dietary glyphosate due to the per capita quantity consumed.

Peer reviewed scientific data abounds about the dangers of glyphosate. There is outright refusal to read these published articles, particularly by those who are supposed to watch out for our health – this is a difficult thing to most people to believe. However, until you are willing to reject the apologists and soothsayers from the food industry and government protective agencies, you're probably not going to be successful losing weight for long. Glyphosate must be removed from your life if you wish to lose weight over the long haul.

There is actually great news about glyphosate. You don't need to be affected by it. Just avoid it. Traditional Caribbean foods are not processed foods. They have almost no grains as the Caribbean carbohydrate starches mostly come from roots, plantains, sweet potatoes and rice (rice has been found at very low levels in glyphosate studies). The traditional Caribbean meat is free range chicken, pork, and goat. Dairy products are a very low percentage of Caribbean foods, and that dairy does not come from the vast grain fed and additive laden system of industrial dairy operations.

Phthalates

"We seem to be accepting as a society that it's acceptable to load up our next generation with chemicals in an unregulated manner and hope they're not bad. We need to change that entire culture."

~ Professor Thomas Zoeller, University of Massachusetts

As a society, it seems that we are all OK with endocrine disruptors. We don't ask and industries don't tell. But phthalates are virulent EDs found in a multitude of common products and absolutely must be avoided.

Many scented items including cosmetics, shampoos, scented skin lotions, and household cleaners are obesogens. These nice smelling chemicals are called phthalates. But exposure to high levels of phthalates has been clearly linked to endocrine disruption, specifically insulin resistance leading to obesity. Of particular concern are shampoos and body cleansers due to their direct contact with moist skin every day. Shampoos are typically made with sodium laureth sulfate, DMDM hydantoin, and dozens of synthetic fragrances. Hair care products and many different skin lotions are noted as a primary phthalate risk, made worse by their application on wet skin with scrubbing into hair follicles.

Scented household sprays are another danger as the droplets of phthalates enter the nasal canal and quickly enter the blood stream. Fresh car scents, bathroom scents, and scented laundry detergent are other sources of phthalates.

Phthalates are EDs that can trigger "death-inducing signaling" in testicular cells, making them die prematurely. Research has linked phthalates to hormone changes, lower sperm count, less mobile sperm, birth defects in the male reproductive system, and thyroid dysfunction. Phthalates are EDs with a direct connection with obesity and diabetes.[16,17]

It's very difficult to avoid these dangerous chemical compounds unless you literally keep a list of them in with you as you shop. They are produced in vast quantities to make plastics malleable. Phthalates are found in food packaging, plastic wrap, vinyl toys, and many more plastic products.

However, they are also found in nail polish, perfume, hair spray. In fact, the cosmetic, hair, and beauty items commonly used are a serious problem that shows up in abdominal fat. Use your due diligence; study the ingredients in your favorite cleansers, shampoos, fragrances, and the plastics around you. Shop for items whose label states, "phthalate-free".

More EDs from industrial chemicals

Atrazine: The atrazine week killer website proudly states that this widely used herbicide is "Safe for people, good for the environment and economy." Many well respected scientists differ, point out the serious endocrine damage from Atrazine.[18] Atrazine is the infamous herbicide that increases estrogen in animals such that male frogs in atrazine waters become "feminized" and produce eggs and have offspring.[19,20] This ED is the go-to herbicide for corn and sugar cane, used on 13.9 million acres of corn and .9 million acres of sugarcane fields each year. The water runoff is pervasive from atrazine is found in drinking water in the majority of continental US and Hawaii.

Organophosphates (OPs): Neurotoxic organophosphate compounds are pesticides that attack the nervous system of insects. They have serious ED damaging effects on testosterone and alter thyroid levels.[21] Even minute exposure to widely used organophosphate pesticides Malathion and Parathion alter hormone function.[22] These pesticides are of particular damage to thyroid function, with the result showing in weight gain. OPs are commonly applied to blueberries, celery, green beans, peaches, and especially to strawberries.

Xenoestrogens: Plastic water bottles, plastic food containers, plastic "food safety" wrap, plus a large number of processed food additives are made with xenoestrogens. Heat and sunlight release dangerous bisphenol A (BPA) from the plastic containers into the liquid. These form a unique family of EDs that imitate the action of estrogen. The critical rise of estrogen levels from xenoestrogens lead to obesity, breast cancer, prostate cancer and testicular cancer.

Phytoestrogens: These are ED's that are linked to low thyroid hormone levels causing thyroid T3 function to be seriously disrupted.[23] Soy is the primary source of phytoestrogens, mimicking and disrupting the action of estrogen. It is believed that the toxic buildup of phytoestrogens form a major source widespread feeling of fatigue and symptoms of low thyroid.[24]

Organochlorine: These ED pesticides are widely applied to apples, tomatoes, russet potatoes, vegetables, and cereal grains. Popular insecticides such as endosulfan, chlordecone, DDT derivatives, and others are part of this ED family. It has been found to significantly disrupt estrogen balance as well as cause reproductive damage.[25] Banned throughout the European Union, Australia, Brazil and other regions of the world, organochlorine is still widely used in the US.

Dioxin: Exposure to this ED typically comes from CAFO meat and farmed fish consumption, along with non-organic dairy and butter. This ED can disrupt the delicate ways both male and female sex hormone signaling occurs leading to weight gain.[26] The SAD gets 93% of its dioxin exposure from meat and dairy products, with very high dioxin coming from commercial dairy.

Perfluorinated chemicals (PFCs): These are obesogens to be strictly avoided but used in such a wide range of products it is difficult to know how to avoid them. They are used to make non-stick cookware, sandwich wrappers, camping tents, carpeting and carpet treatments. The specific way they cause obesity is that they cause serious thyroid hormonal disorders.[27,28]

Beauty product endocrine disruptors

What you put on your skin can make you fat. According to *safecosmetics.org*, the average woman puts roughly 500 chemicals on her body each day provided by the beauty industry that uses over 10,000 chemicals into their products. Many of these are confirmed EDs. It is estimated that 60% of the creams, lotions, shampoos, and fragrance are absorbed where they enter the bloodstream and travel to the brain.

Packaging cosmetic products cleverly hides most of the worst ingredients so much that it is difficult to tell without researching each individual product. The language and ingredient descriptions are purposely vague. The four categories of ED cosmetics are parabens, phthalates, pesticides, and plastics. Do your research so you know what to buy.

Fragrances, mostly come from petroleum distillates.
Parabens, made up of multiple anti-bacterial agents and preservatives in cosmetics.
Phthalates, plastic containers of cosmetics leach into the lotion.
Sodium lauryl sulfate, widely used in shampoos.
Triethanolamine, a pH balancing agent that acts as a surfactant.
Triclosan, an antimicrobial compound in deodorant and hand sanitizers.
Coloring agents, such as hair dye, eye shadow, eye liner, lipstick.

Lose weight despite the chemical invaders

The worst result of this information would be to panic and just give up; to claim that there is no way to avoid the endocrine disruptors that surround us. However, the system you are reading is the Carefree Caribbean Weightloss system. The message should be clear. Relax and trust yourself that everything will be OK.

There is an attitude adjustment needed throughout the Carefree system. Nowhere is the change in attitude needed more than in countering the chemical invasion of your environment, foods, and cosmetics. You won't succeed unless you actively work to avoid contact with the synthetic chemicals that harm you. However, you won't succeed if you let your fears take over your life and live in even more stress.

Oddly enough, the act of being carefree will get you through the morass. While others suffer from stress and indecision, you should have learned by now how to have a bite of dark chocolate and come up with a simple solution. Walk barefoot, sing to your new favorite songs, laugh more. Get rid of the problems little by little and then don't stress yourself about it.

You can easily avoid the toxic onslaught in cosmetics. There are many cosmetics that feature safe, non ED ingredients. They are easy to buy online, prices similar to what you may pay now, and perform considerably better than the chemical lab experiment you smear on yourself every day. You'll probably never find a way to get 100% pure cosmetic products, shampoos, fragrances, and nail polish. But with a plan of action, you'll easily avoid the worst culprit, uneducated buying habits.

How to avoid endocrine disruptors

Because of the enormous amount of toxic chemical around you, it's impossible to live "toxin free." However, you can significantly limit your exposure by following some basic guidelines:

1. Choose food grown fresh or organic. Processed and packaged items are usually loaded with toxic chemicals. Follow the EWG guidelines in choosing food to buy.
2. Eat free range meats, dairy, butter, and eggs to limit the intake of toxins. Avoid processed meats, deli meats, processed cheese, standard yogurt, and standard ice cream.
3. Eat seafood that has an EWG safe rating. Select seafood with the highest omega-3 fatty acids then also take w a high quality fish oil.
4. Avoid canned foods and plastic containers; instead get glass bottles or frozen foods after carefully reading labels.
5. Refrigerate or freeze food in glass, not plastic. Never warm food in plastic container. Get rid of plastic wrap; just use wax paper instead.
6. Cook in cast iron, glass, ceramic pots and pans. Get rid of everything that has a non-stick surface, never cook in aluminum, and use wooden spatulas and spoons.
7. Install a high quality water filter for your tap water. Be sure filter is changed frequently. Avoid plastic water bottles, use glass instead.
8. Buy organic shampoo, deodorant, cosmetics, and toothpaste. Use EWG's Skin Deep database to choose personal care item.

Eight

THE BALANCE OF EXERCISE

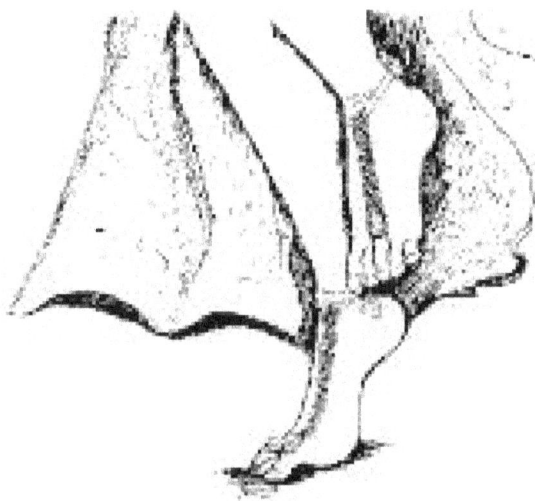

"Practicing balance teaches us what we can control, what we can't yet control, and how badly we lose control when things don't go the way we want."
~ Nellie Vladimirovna Kim, Olympic Gymnastics Champion

It's clear that the endocrine system is where your weightloss focus should be. Hormones tell your body what to do including what to burn for energy, what to store as fat, and even what your mood will be. By focusing on your endocrine system, you can learn to manipulate hormonal release by what you eat, how much stress you have, and how active you are. This is the role of exercise – how to use exercise to manipulate your hormones to help you.

Here is where the Caribbean Sea can alter your life once again. Island culture features an active physical life filled with hard work, healthful food, and a stress free way of living that makes the right hormonal manipulation choices for you. The Caribbean attitude is the key for you to lose weight permanently, if you will let this attitude out of its cage. This attitude also is an important part of the way you move about.

A strenuous, active life is a key player in manipulating hormones to work for you. Used wisely, regular strenuous activity lasting about half an hour triggers hormones to lead the weightloss process, even triggering adrenalin, HGH, and testosterone, while at the same time reducing cortisol. Importantly, the right exercise and the right timing of exercise also triggers hormones by the positive mood created, extending feel-good hormones.

Enough is enough

There is a fine line between strenuous exercise and overly strenuous exercise. This line is entirely personal; the difference between enough and too much varies greatly from person to person. But when it comes to hormone manipulation, exercise should have a new objective. No longer should you be concerned with sweating off pounds or building muscles, but instead focus on triggering favorable hormonal response.

With excessive exercise, cortisol levels skyrocket and nullify the effect from feel-good hormones. For adults seeking weightloss, it's important to avoid excessive exercise as this can also lead to hypothyroidism. One of the worst outcomes would be adrenal fatigue which can result from too much cardiovascular training.

For adults, clearly the most popular form of exercise is steady-state cardio training. Running at the same steady pace for an hour or more, swimming at a steady pace, bicycling at a steady pace, and using a stair climber at a gym are each problematic for adult weightloss.

You'll also see this described as chronic cardio. It is found in excessive aerobic exercise where the elapsed time of the activity is of great importance. At 45 minutes your mental alarm bell should sound that it's time to shut things down. A long workout of continuous cardiovascular stress causes a series of biochemical reactions leading to dreaded hormonal reactions.

Excessive training, often called overtraining, is age regulated. This means that the hours or miles of training done at age 25 has a different hormonal effect on the body as the same workload done at age 50, no matter if it seems harder or easier at age 50. As we age, the body interprets stress differently than it did in our 20's, more cortisol is released with higher workloads at age 50 than at age 25. Overtraining should be seen as something to avoid. No training at all should be seen as something to avoid. Consequently, you need to be on the lookout for your personal sweet spot.

Cortisol rears its ugly head

Exercise should be your time to get away from it all; your free time to decompress. You should feel freedom from all the pressures driving you crazy as you get ready for your workout. However, you should also be aware that exercise must be manipulated to work for you, not against you. Even what you do getting ready to exercise is of great importance in controlling cortisol.

One key problem of overtraining as an adult is the way it negatively affects sleep, both duration of sleep and quality of sleep. Both of these sleep problems add to even more hormonal disruption, particularly cortisol release. Great effort should be spent on getting highest quality sleep.

Obviously, then, the effort to lose weight and shape yourself isn't simply a matter of diet and exercise, but how to limit and control stress in the process of normal daily life. Choking off of the release of cortisol and its mischievous partner in crime, estrogen, comes as a result of relaxation, assuming you are taking in the right nutrients at the right time. Relaxing, sleeping, laughing and playing thus become the top four "to do" objectives for each day to control. Therefore, find a way to have exercise make you laugh, literally. Play more the way you used to do on the school playground. Afterwards, watch stupid movies that make you laugh, fewer intellectually stimulating ones. This is a way to manipulate cortisol.

Consistency is a key to the entire Carefree Caribbean Weightloss system. In terms of developing the habit of exercising most days, make up your mind on a time of day that you'll stick with. Your internal clock should point to that time as something to look forward to, not something to dread. If you dread your workouts, something is wrong and you need to change what you do. Brisk walking is a great starting point.

There are many physical actions you can do to voluntarily trigger a hormonal surge that aids you. When you consciously blend the physical activity with a mental one, the triggering effect is greatly enhanced. For example, consider the mind/body activity you can do with strength and confidence before your workout.

Research out of Harvard supports this. In this study, researcher Amy Cuddy found that simply holding your arms up like in the Rocky movie in "high-power" poses for about two minutes triggers the release of 20% more testosterone while reducing cortisol by about 25% for both women and men.[1] This means as you are getting ready to exercise, take a couple of minutes before you start to stand and relax. Breathe deeply as you go into your Rocky pose, which will look like a warmup stretch to onlookers. Just like that, you'll voluntarily manipulate hormones.

Next, start your workout with a few minutes of balance oriented exercises. All you need to do is to practice balance activities while focusing on control of your body. You'll aid your positive hormonal releases while limiting the negative ones. You get much more than simply contracting muscles and sweating; you actually teach yourself body control. Furthermore, if your exercise program is specifically designed to be interesting, fun, entertaining, then you have an even better chance of success. Like cats, humans are curious about interesting things.

Landing squarely on your feet

Your exercise should complement your efforts at relaxation, not run counter to it. This is why the entire Caribbean Weightloss system emphasizes balance training. Something happens to us as we focus on balance, something way beyond flexing muscles. If you are thrust out of balance, you instantly and automatically enter a mental state of total focus on not falling on your butt. This focus overwhelms you until you regain control.

During these moments of calm concentration on body control, cortisol is choked off. Researchers found that four months of regular "mindfulness training" that included balance oriented yoga-like exercise resulted in loss in body fat among overweight and obese women.[2] Balance and it's unique connection of physical and mental is where your exercise should be.

Regularly practiced activities that challenge your balance strengthen, challenge, invigorate, and leave you relaxed when you're done. Spend the first five minutes balancing so that the rest of your exercise time will be influenced by those few focused minutes. In this way you manipulate cortisol as well as serotonin secretions.

When you fight to control your equilibrium, you engage the neuromuscular process known as proprioception. In effect, as you lean too far to the right, tiny muscles around joints instantly fire on the left side – you can even see them jiggle as they contract. This is how you correct your balance without ever once thinking about it. This happens over and over in the silent battle to stand upright.

Importantly, balance involves the brain – you have to concentrate or you fall. It isn't that you have to think "fire the left side! No, fire the right side! Oops, back to the left side!" That automatic balancing happens best if you find a mental zone of calm control. Sometimes you wind up concentrating so hard on staying under control that you are oblivious to surroundings, to the sounds, to the sights, and to any feelings you may have. This is total focus on standing up to control yourself or you fall.

In this strange mental/physical state of maintaining balance you manipulate your hormones. Cortisol is choked off by balance activity. Yoga masters know this state very well. Tai Chi masters know this state. The deep breathing and concentration of Buddhist monks know this state. This is where body control controls the mind.

All you need is to teach yourself to get into the mental zone of calmness, then concentrate in your half hour of exercise – no distractions, please. Just wiggling to keep from falling does the job of emptying your brain of all stress and worry. The workout itself, not the muscles or reps or sweat droplets, will become part of your hormone manipulation process. It's interesting. It's easy. It's fun. It will help you lose weight and look better.

One aspect of balance training that is of particular value to weightloss is exercising barefoot as often as you can. The mass of 200,000 neurosensors in the feet are stimulated when you go barefoot; they are genetically programmed to respond to the ground. After four million years of cultivating the foot's ability to read the surface of the ground, modern man has dulled this fabulous sensory device, the foot. Although we cover the feet with shoes, we don't remove the neurosensors.

It's not hard to do, but it is often hard to accept the benefits of exercising barefoot. Once you clear your brain of doubts and self-destructive thoughts, getting barefoot for exercise can trigger unknown sensations.

A report in the *Journal of Alternative and Complementary Medicine* confirmed that walking or exercising barefoot aids in normalizing daily cortisol rhythm and improves sleep.[3] There is evidence that the electric charge from the core of earth connects at the bare foot to calm us, relax us, and bring about anti-inflammation. A peer reviewed study in 2004 found that cortisol levels were reduced by contacting the foot to ground during sleep.[4]

Ask yourself why walking barefoot on the beach is such an intoxicating thing to do? Why does walking barefoot in the grass seem so invigorating? Is it possible that there is something beyond muscles and force put on the ground, something of an electric connection happening as the foot contacts the earth? The research definitely sides with the electric grounding narrative.[5]

Stepping on a banana peel

Imagine that you have a big bag of groceries in your arms as you walk and suddenly you step on a banana peel. Something instantly takes over your body, and rather than sprawling on your butt, you somehow manage to fall gracefully, groceries intact. No injuries, no spilt groceries, and onlookers amazed at how cool you responded. This is the realm of kinesthetic awareness, the technical term for body control in motion. It is the feel for (awareness) of your center of mass, or the way that humans take control of planned and unplanned movements.

A cat doesn't need a college course on kinesthetic awareness to land on four feet after a fall, it's built-in. The same is true for humans. Some people are born with a lot of athletic body control, others not so much. But humans are born with a very big brain, and if you practice at it, this brain can teach the body remarkable control of movement and balance.

By focusing on body control, not only do you keep your balance, but you teach yourself to control your life. This isn't some voodoo or deep psychological analysis, it is simple habit building. Every day you spend a few minutes to practice the habit of balance or controlling yourself. You get used to surrounding yourself with balance, so much that you become very aware of the sensation of being out of balance. You become aware of where you are in relation to the pull of gravity.

Gravity doesn't change. Your mass doesn't change. But you change the way you perceive it. This will cost you nothing but a few minutes of your time. Go ahead, start now teaching yourself to walk around the house with a big book balanced on your head. Stand on one foot, then the other, go up the stairs then stoop down to touch the ground. This may seem stupid, but it is very, very hard to do and it teaches body control.

Kinesthetic awareness provides a step-by-step way to improve body control, and if you'll allow it, this leads to higher levels of satisfaction, better mood, and better shape. This is movement sense, and the way the brain integrates proprioceptive input with vestibular input (inner ear balancing sense.)

Don't get too caught up into the science of it all. When you do the exercises, you'll manipulate your cortisol levels down if you believe the science of it or not. Just let yourself enjoy development of better balance and body control. Focus on really having fun.

Islanders regularly practice balance without giving it much thought. Balance and body control are at the core of Caribbean life. Generations of Islanders developed very high levels of balance as they worked the small fishing boats that rocked in the sea. This region of earth is where you find women who sell fruit from a basket balanced on their head. The limited amount of labor-saving tools in traditional Caribbean society means that Islanders often work in construction or road work that requires tremendous body control.

And then there is dance. You'll see little girls salsa dancing with amazing rhythm and body control, just as you'll see great dancing by elderly couples. Dance seems to be part of the DNA of Islanders. Dancing to the popular songs of the Caribbean is as much a part of life as sand, sunshine, and *sofrito*. Dance is frequently blended with rum, wine, and drinks of all kinds. In the Caribbean, dance is a big part of the region's culture.

However, dance also teaches body control, and body control teaches relaxation. It's almost like the adage, "what came first, the chicken or the egg." For you, accept the fact that physical balance, kinesthetic awareness and coordination are highly prevalent in traditional Caribbean life. It is Caribbean lifestyle that will guide you through your journey to a thinner you. These qualities are woven into the Carefree Caribbean Weightloss system.

Life in balance

"Life is like riding a bicycle. To keep your balance, you must keep moving."
   ~ Albert Einstein

It doesn't take much to improve your balance, and the exercises don't need to be particularly difficult, but some of them can be quite difficult. You don't need equipment or a special place, the grass or your carpet work great. A box, a few tennis balls, a playground ball, a broomstick, and a few other simple tools will all help keep the workouts interesting.

The hardest part about balance training is the attitude adjustment. The exercises are weird, different, unique, sometimes hard for onlookers to figure out what the hell is going on. Your job is to be you, just a person doing something different. Step up and be bold, walk on tennis balls. Get a playground ball and roll it with your shin. Balance a broomstick.

Recent studies point to the quick-learning aspect of balance training. Researchers have found considerable improvement in subjects evaluated on multiple balance tests in 11 to 12 weeks of moderate but consistent work at balance exercises.[6] This means that you'll never get bored; it's exhilarating to get better week to week. Your skills at body control rapidly improve and you're constantly trying new challenges to test yourself. This makes it a lot of fun.

Exercising with a park bench, a box or a sturdy milkcrate is an excellent way to stress balance on one foot as you squat down or lift your leg up. There are a dozen bench or box exercises you can do that force you to concentrate on balance as you resist against gravity. Some are easy, some are embarrassingly hard. Many of the exercises are almost like games where you don't count sets and reps. Some of the more strenuous ones work best at two sets of six to eight repetitions per leg (see Chapter 10). You'll find that a good sturdy milk crate has multiple benefits, as you exercise stepping on and off, sitting on, leaning on, as well as keeping your exercise equipment in it. They are easy to carry your exercise tools (toys) to a field or into a room or in the trunk of your car.

Proprioception

"Humans don't have a single organ or body part for proprioception. The job is done by the entire nervous system working as a whole. From muscles and joints messages are sent to the spinal cord and on to the brain. The brain instantly decides what to do and messages those muscles and joints with instructions, repeated again and again."

~ Nellie Vladimirovna Kim, Olympic Gymnastics Champion

One of the most successful activities for weightloss is yoga. There are many elements of yoga – not all – that are similar to the balance based exercise that is so essential to the Carefree system. Yoga puts great emphasis on body control, mostly from stationary poses.

However, it is the movement in balance stressing component of yoga activities that have received most scientific inquiry, not the stationary poses. Studies have reported that specific yoga activities are beneficial in weightloss programs, specifically in improving body composition.[7]

Balance training exercises provide sensory input to stay focused, and thus train the body to be more alert throughout the day to sensory influences. These stabilizing activities of balance have been found to aid a nervous system that has become overly aroused by stress, fear, deadlines, frustration, anger, etc.

But balance needs to go to the next level, a body in motion. Furthermore, when performing difficult exercises such as sitting down on a bench and getting back up, all on one leg, the activity is considered resistance training. Body weight can be a very, very heavy object to lift when the position or body angle makes the action hard to do. Therefore, when you do balance oriented training you simultaneously do resistance training on many of the exercises.

Proprioceptive exercise is often misunderstood to be something done on an unstable surface in an effort to develop joint stability. This isn't the case as most of the work in the Carefree system, though not all, is done on flat ground. Fighting for balance while standing on the ground is the constant communication throughout your nervous system messaging the brain how you're holding up in your environment. It is the ability to sense body control in very simple exercises, to move freely and instantly without thinking about what to do.

Hopefully, you haven't had a proprioceptive test recently, as the most common test is the police field sobriety to test for drunk drivers. But if you took the test it would be easy because your proprioceptive skills would be outstanding. With five minutes of effort most days, you can get proprioception development, and in the process make a connection of brain and body, something of extreme importance to weightloss.[8,9] By incorporating proprioception into your exercise routine you double the benefits in the same amount of time.

A series of simple balance and balance with resistance exercises hone your "sixth sense" which is known to be proprioception. This is more than just a sense or skill, it is woven into the fabric of the survival of the fittest.

From chaos to taking control

Once you appreciate the importance of taking control of your body as it stands and as it moves, a bunch of silly balancing exercises change into something more substantial. You'll quickly notice that the physical process of body control does something to your mental process whether you try to or not. Proprioception is your way to practice changing chaos into control.

Proprioceptive sensations (the readings we get from joints, connective tissues, and muscles) are found by a wide variety of activities ranging from body weight exercises to hard-to-lift weights. By focusing on the movements, especially those that require the foot to play an active part of providing a firm base on the ground, balance oriented exercises stimulate the proprioceptive senses. This is how humans evolved.

These exercises that calm you and alert your attention can be fun, interesting, and when you want, extremely difficult. Want to try something very difficult to challenge your body control? Without touching ground, try to walk a line of half a dozen tennis balls placed a foot apart, then turn around and walk back.

It is the carryover that balance oriented exercises bring to you throughout the day, as well as your strong feeling of control that make proprioceptive exercises so important to weightloss.[10] All of this adds up to making a conscious effort to connect the brain and the body during exercise. It doesn't take much, but it does require consistent challenge to your balance. Whatever you do, don't overthink this. It's like playing.

Before any workout, begin with dynamic flexibility exercises which warm you, stretch you, and develop your balance all in one activity. If your favorite exercise is jogging, it is easy as warming up by skipping to the front, then to the side for a while. If it is weight lifting you enjoy, it is easy to train with suspension cords (TRX) balancing on one foot that put great stress on proprioception. If you have almost no time due to long days at work, half an hour of balance oriented training is easy to do in your apartment, back yard, or garage.

The effort is a constant but modest stress on muscles, especially if you do multi-tasking such as keeping balance while walking sideways on a curb or walking up a flight of stairs while balancing a dictionary on your head. Your feet, glutes, hips and abs will get sore even though not one exercise will be done targeting these muscles.

Balance oriented exercise is the opposite of brute force exercise. It is a blend of calm relaxation with moments of very mentally exhausting, stimulating, and focusing times. Memory is sharpened, creativity is enhanced. There is a direct result in reducing depression and improving cognition. In comparison, researchers have found that increasing cardiovascular fitness fails to bring beneficial effects cognition.[11] It is balance training that stimulates memory and spatial cognition. As you start out it can be quite challenging, frustrating, embarrassing, and painful. It can also be a hell of a lot of fun. You get to pick and choose.

Getting started

"Man cannot discover new oceans unless he has the courage to lose sight of the shore."
   ~ Andre Gide

If you go to a major league baseball pre game warmup, you'll be surprised to see the many of the players doing a strange series of dance-like exercises for warmup. Top track athletes, lots of elite soccer stars, and all of the adults who work with me do skips, leg swings, dips, and strange walks. These motions are known as dynamic flexibility, which are dance-like, with sweeping motions. They warm, stretch, and develop your ability to control motions. They can be easy, or they can be very hard to do until you develop some skill. Challenge yourself, get good at doing these.

Dynamic flexibility is a great way to start. In that balance is interwoven with the dynamic flexibility motions, you get two for one.

Some balance oriented exercises to choose from:

Dynamic Flexibility
Skipping, to front, sideways, backwards
Walking, right knee lifted up to left elbow
Grab foot behind you as you squat
Standing, lift leg parallel to ground front, side, back
Leg swings, front to back, then left to right

Bodyweight exercises
Pistol squats (touch butt on box while one foot extended in front)
Lunges to front, side, back, then a ¾ turn and lunge
Low walks (walk with hips low, dragging back foot from back to front)
Spiderman (kneel raising left leg straight back right arm straight front)

Playground ball exercises
Kneeling, put rear shin on ball then roll front to back
Ball against wall, back touching ball, back squats
Ball against wall, back touching ball, back squats with one leg
Single leg squat, touches knee to ball on ground

Tennis balls
Stand on two tennis balls
Stand on one tennis ball
Walk a line of 6 tennis balls, turn and walk back
Tap ball between feet like soccer ball

Jumps
Knees to chest jumps
Jump over broomstick that rests on milk crate
Lunge position jumps
Short hops (50 fast one foot hops completed in 10 yards)

Dumbbells
Boxer shadow punching (light dumbbells)
Falling lunge on to box

Russian dead lifts (weight in right bend to touch left toe)
Rowing while kneeling from box or bench
Step ups

Bulgarian sandbag exercises
Swing bag between legs up and back
Squat with bag on shoulders
Squat jumps with bag on shoulders
On shoulder lunge to front, side, back
Turkish get ups, lie with bag on shoulder and get up

Suspension cords (TRX)
At 45° angle pull up, legs spread on ground
At 45° angle pull up, single leg on ground
Push up, legs spread on ground
Overhead arches lunge, hips gently move down and back

Box drills (milk crates)
Stand one foot on box, touch ground with other heel and back up
Hands on box, belly up, straight leg lift
Hands on box, belly down, straight leg lift
Sit on box, knees to chest
Stand, 2 feet on ground, squat till butt touches box
Stand, 1 foot on ground, squat till butt touches box

Broomstick
Balance stick in hand
Balance stick in hand on one foot
Jump side to side over stick lying at 45°
Lunge forward, 2 hands holding stick, plant stick to side like flagpole

Medicine ball
Side heave into wall and catch
Top of head heave into wall and catch
Step and heave for distance
Jump in air and smash onto ground

Optional tools for balance

Choose from milk crates, wobble boards, balance boards, balance discs, Bosu balls, playground ball, medicine balls, tennis balls, broom sticks. Use a curb and a park bench. TRX suspension cords are a great tool for strength, quite difficult to navigate. Some dumbbells work great, a jump rope helps, and a Bulgarian sandbag is tremendous.

You can make a Bulgarian sandbag in 10 minutes. Buy a plastic bag of garden sand, about 35 pounds, don't open the plastic. Put it into a thick plastic garbage bag and tape it shut with packing tape. Put this double bagged weight into a sturdy sausage shaped gym bag. It's that easy.

The best medicine balls are the ones that bounce, as this brings multiple activities you can do with one ball. Weights vary, but 6 to 8 pound balls seem to provide the most variety of exercises.

Tools play an important part in making the entire Carefree system fun. Onlookers will stare, trying to figure what the hell you're doing, let alone why. Balance and body control exercises with playground tools keep you connected with the program: not just diet, not just exercise, not just stress reduction. These tools can become important parts of your overall effort to change your attitude. Become carefree.

Nine

THE MAGIC OF CARIBBEAN COOKING

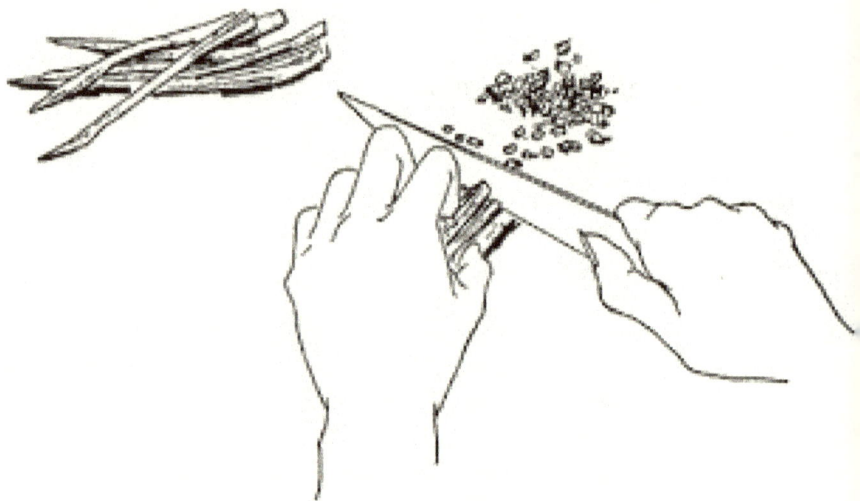

"I cook with wine. Sometimes I even add it to the food."
~ W.C. Fields

Flavor (*Savor*)

Caribbean and Latin meals are very flavorful, multi-layered tastes, unexpected contrasts, and an aroma of the gods. Many dishes start as heating olive oil in a pan, then some garlic, then onion, then bell pepper, then come the herbs and spices. After that it varies between tomato, often carrot, and whatever else that is on hand that might liven up the taste. Measurements are mostly by hand, literally. A pinch of cayenne pepper or salt is universally measured in the palm of the hand, and a cup is an estimate.

Latin foods are frequently made by "sweating" the pan, as a little water is added to steam-heat up the sauté process several times during the preparation. Rarely will you see this style of cooking timed to the minute, it is much more often cooked to see how it looks and how it tastes along the way. The sauces tend to cook a long time for the flavor to mature, then blend with the dish, rather than spooned on at the table. Often the sauces are made in large batches, used and reused, added to and adjusted.

In the small family restaurants that are scattered throughout the Caribbean, not one of the cooks ever went to cooking school, and many never finished high school. Most have never picked up a cookbook in their life, wouldn't know the name Cordon Bleu, Martha Stewart, or a Michelin rating. The one master chef that all cooks pay homage to is...*abuela* (grandmother).

There are literally thousands of Caribbean recipes to choose from. The following have been chosen to fit the guidelines of Carefree Caribbean weightloss. Several traditional recipes have been doctored to avoid problem food choices and replace with somewhat similar but more fitting choices.

It's best to follow the measurements the first time to get a feel for the recipe, after that it's time for you to add or subtract to make it your way. Most important, don't worry if you don't have all the right ingredients. Here again it's mind over matter – I don't mind and it don't matter.

Basic sauces

Sofrito Cubano
2 Tbsp olive oil
4 medium tomatoes, chopped
1 green pepper, chopped
1 small onion, chopped
3 garlic cloves, chopped
½ tsp cumin
½ tsp oregano
1 tsp sea salt (when done)
½ tsp pepper (fresh ground)

Heat oil in saucepan, hot but not smoking.
Sauté all in hot oil until vegetables are limp.
Refrigerate remainder, use as needed.

Hogao (Colombian Creole Sauce)
3 Tbsp coconut oil
3 medium tomatoes, chopped
½ cup chopped onions
1 garlic clove, minced
1 tsp cumin
Sea salt and pepper to taste
Heat oil in saucepan, sauté garlic 2 min.
Add tomatoes, onions and cumin, sauté 10 min.
Reduce heat, add salt & pepper, cook 5 minutes until it thickens.

Salsa Tomato
10 medium tomatoes, diced
3 garlic cloves, minced
1 onion, chopped
½ cup tomato sauce
½ cup cilantro, coarsely chopped
¼ cup jalapeno (hot) or Anaheim (mild) chili, finely chopped
2 Tbsp honey
1 Tbsp sea salt
1 ½ tsp cumin
Mix with spoon in bowl or briefly blend in blender.

Mayonnaise Espanola
1 cup olive oil (mild or coconut oil)
1 egg yolk (room temperature)
1 Tbsp lemon or lime juice
¾ tsp sea salt
½ tsp dry mustard
¼ tsp fresh ground pepper
In blender put egg, juice, spices and ¼ of the oil, blend 10 sec.
Slowly drizzle remaining ¾ oil, stop for 20 seconds, then again.

Guacamole

2 avocados, large, peeled, 1 mashed the other finely chopped.
2 limes, juiced
1 medium tomato, finely chopped
¼ cup onion, very finely minced
¼ cup jalapeno or mild chili, finely chopped
¼ cup cilantro, finely chopped
¼ tsp sea salt
¼ tsp cumin
¼ tsp chili powder (hot) or paprika (mild)

Put tomatoes in large bowl, pour boiling water over 30 sec.
Drain water, cover with cold water, then peel off skins.
Add avocados, lime juice, mix all ingredients except cilantro.
Put on serving dish, add cilantro on top.

Balsamic Vinaigrette

½ cup olive oil
¼ cup balsamic vinegar
1 Tbsp Italian seasoning

Add all to glass cruet, shake, pour.

Jamaican Jerk Sauce

4 garlic cloves, minced
2 limes juiced
2 Tbsp olive oil
½ cup sliced scallions
½ cup minced onion
1 Tbsp honey
1 tsp cayenne powder (hot) or paprika (mild)
1 tsp cinnamon
1 tsp thyme
1 tsp black pepper
1 tsp sea salt
½ tsp nutmeg
½ tsp allspice
½ tsp ginger

Blend all, refrigerate what you don't use.

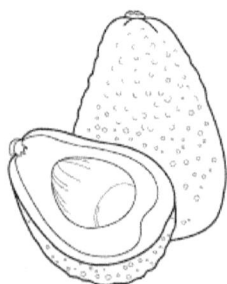

Avocados are a major part of the Caribbean diet, eaten at almost every meal. The fats and nutrients are of extreme help in weightloss.

Molé de Pollo (Mexican chocolate chicken)

2 lbs chicken thighs, boneless, skinless
¼ tsp sea salt, divided
Pinch black pepper
2 Tbsp coconut oil, divided
3 cloves garlic, minced
1 Tbsp chili powder
¼ tsp cumin
½ tsp cinnamon
1 cup tomato sauce
½ cup chicken broth
¼ cup semisweet chocolate
1 Tbsp almond butter
1 Tbsp toasted sesame seeds

Season chicken with pepper and half the salt.
Heat 1/2 oil in frypan at med high, brown chicken 4 min ea side.
Reduce heat, add oil, garlic, chili, cumin, cinnamon, salt.
Sautee 30 sec, add tomato sauce, broth, chocolate, almond.
Simmer and stir, add chicken + juices.
Simmer all 10 min. Serve sprinkled with sesame seeds.

Salsa Parrilla (Latin barbeque sauce)

2 cloves garlic, minced
1 onion, minced
2 Tbsp olive oil
1 can tomato paste, 6 oz
2 cups tomatoes, diced
2 Tbsp honey

2 Tbsp balsamic vinegar
1 cup water, added if needed
1 Tbsp Dijon mustard
½ tsp paprika
½ tsp oregano
¼ tsp pepper
¼ tsp cayenne
½ tsp sea salt to taste
Heat oil in saucepan to medium, sauté garlic and onion 4 min.
Reduce heat to medium low, stir in tomato paste, then sauté tomatoes.
Add water as needed, honey, mustard, spices.
Simmer 20 minutes.

Side Dishes

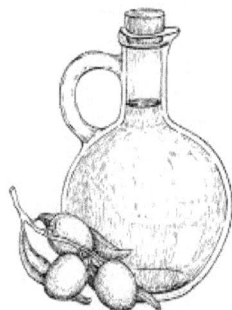

Plan on buying and using a lot of olive oil. For mayonnaise, use mild olive oil. The rest of the time go for the hard stuff, cold pressed extra virgin.

Curtido (Salvadorian sauerkraut)
2 heads cabbage, thinly sliced
3 carrots, grated
2 peppers, jalapeno (hot) or Anaheim (mild), cored and diced
1 onion, thinly sliced
3 Tbsp sea salt
1 Tbsp oregano
Put cabbage in hot water 15 seconds, drain and dry.
Mix everything but salt in very large bowl.
Sprinkle in salt, mix, pound and press in towel 10 min.
Put in large airlock jars, press down veggies, leave 2" brine on top.
Seal jars, store in dark 2 weeks or longer.

Mexican Pan de Elote (corn bread)

1 red bell pepper, cored and chopped
¾ cup harina (cornmeal)
½ cup Greek yogurt
2 eggs
2 cups corn kernels (canned is OK)
1 – 2 cups water (add as needed)
4 Tbsp coconut oil
1 tsp paprika
¼ tsp cayenne
1 tsp baking powder
1 tsp sea salt

Preheat oven @ 400F with large frypan in middle rack.
In large bowl, beat eggs, yogurt, oil, ½ oil, ½ cup water.
Mix harina, baking powder, then mix in red pepper, corn, and spices.
Remove hot frypan from oven, add remaining oil. (Careful, hot!)
Return frypan to oven 10 min until oil is very hot.
Add corn mixture, bake 20 – 25 min till top is golden brown.
Serve immediately, still very hot.

Flatbreads

Faina (garbanzo flatbread)

2 ½ cups garbanzo bean flour
2 cups water
2 Tbsp olive oil (for the flatbread)
2 Tbsp coconut oil (for the pan)
¾ tsp sea salt
¼ tsp pepper

Whisk flour with spices and olive oil.
Whisk in 1 ¾ cup water.
Set aside 30 min for absorption.
Preheat oven @ 450F, then add pizza pan for 5 min.
Add coconut oil to pizza pan, return to oven for 3 min.
Add remaining water to flour, mix, pour evenly on hot pan.
Bake 15 min for flatbread, 30 min if you want it crispy.
Serve when it is hot, hot, hot.

Pan de Arroz (rice cakes)
1 cup leftover rice, well packed
1 egg, beaten
1 Tbsp olive oil
Sea salt and pepper to taste
Mix rice, egg, and spices in large bowl, place in freezer 20 min.
Heat frypan on medium-low 10 min, add oil, return to heat.
Form mixture into golf ball sizes, place on frypan, press into discs.
Cook 5 – 8 min each side, remove from heat to paper towel on plate.

Cassava Flatbread
2 cups cassava flour
1 cup Greek yogurt
½ cup olive oil (divided)
½ cup water
1 tsp sea salt
Pepper to taste
In large bowl mix ingredients and ½ oil until dough is smooth.
Heat frypan to medium low, add oil a little at a time.
Form dough into 10 golf balls, press into discs on frypan.
Cook 2 or 3 min each side.

Trini Roti (sweet potato flatbread)
1 cup mashed sweet potato, steamed, peeled, then mashed
1 cup cassava flour for mixing (can substitute cornmeal)
½ cup cassava flour for dusting hands and cutting board
1 – 2 cups water, added a little at t time as needed
Mix all in large bowl, don't kneed more than minimum.
Roll into log on cutting board dusted with flour.
Cut into 3 even parts.
Make into golf ball with hands dusted with flour.
Flatten into disc, use roller to make into tortilla sized disc.
Heat large fry pan on medium low, cook one disc at a time.
Turn over every 20 – 30 seconds for about 3 min.
Remove from heat, let settle on tea towel.

Wake up (*Despierta!*)

Tortilla Puertoriquena
4 eggs, lightly beaten
3 Tbsp olive oil
1 plantain, boiled, sliced into ½ inch chips
1 avocado, sliced, for garnish
½ cup sliced pork leftovers
Sea salt, pepper to taste
Fry plantain chips in 1 Tbsp oil about 4 minutes on med.
Add pork, cook 2 min, then put pork and plantains on paper towels.
Reduce heat, pour in eggs.
After 2 minutes, add pork and plantains for another min.
Flip over to cook other side about 2 min.

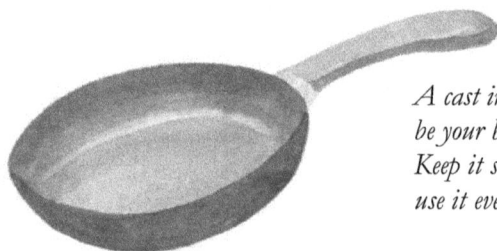

A cast iron sauté pan will be your best kitchen tool. Keep it seasoned and you'll use it every day.

Spanish Omelet
2 eggs
1 Tbsp onion, diced
1 Tbsp tomato, diced
1 Tbsp coconut oil
Sea salt, pepper to taste
Heat iron frypan on medium until drop of water sizzles.
Add oil, make sure it covers frypan.
Sautee onion and tomato 2 min.
Moderately beat eggs, add to pan.
Cook at medium heat until top almost done.
Fold ½ eggs on top of other half.
Cook 30 seconds, then slide to plate.

Huevos con Yuca (fried eggs and yuca)

2 eggs
1 Tbsp tomato, diced
½ cup leftover boiled yuca, diced
½ cup sofrito
¼ cup green olives, diced
1 Tbsp olive oil
Sea salt, pepper to taste
Preheat frypan, then add oil to spread around pan.
Sauté yuca, tomatoes, *sofrito* and olives, set aside.
Fry eggs, yolks up, put on top of sautéed yuca and vegetables.

Baked egg avocado

2 eggs
1 avocado, halved, pitted, scoop out spoonful of each hole.
Sea salt to taste
Pepper to taste
Preheat oven @ 425F.
Cut off ½" of avocado crown so it sits flat with scoop side up.
Put on baking pan, sprinkle salt and pepper into each hole.
Whisk eggs, add salt and pepper, pour into avocado holes.
Bake 15 to 18 min until eggs fully cooked.

Arepas

2 cups water
1 ½ cup harina PAN (pre-cooked white corn meal)
1 tsp sea salt
1 tsp olive oil
Mix water and salt until dissolved in medium bowl.
Slowly add harina, mix with hands to break lumps.
Let mixture rest 5 min, preheat large iron frypan on med.
Add oil to mixture, blend with hands 2 min until dough is formed.
Make golf ball sized dough, flatten until ½" thick discs.
Fry discs 5 – 7 min until both sides are golden brown.
Serve hot, cut each in middle to make 2 discs on plate.
Fill with egg, chicken, pork, cheese, whatever you have.

Tortilla Espanola (Spanish roast eggs and potatoes)

6 eggs
4 red potatoes, peeled, diced
4 Tbsp olive oil, divided
1 onion, sliced
1 red bell pepper, long thin slices
¼ cup cilantro
Sea salt and pepper to taste

Heat ½ oil in large frypan medium low.
Cook potatoes turning regularly until tender, 20+ min.
Remove potatoes to bowl, mix in salt, pepper.
Heat ½ oil on medium, sauté onions, red peppers 8 min.
Put in separate bowl.
Whisk eggs in large bowl, stir in onions, potatoes, peppers.
Heat remaining oil at med low, add eggs until bottom begins to brown.
Cover frypan, turn upside down, allow eggs to fall on to cover.
Return eggs to frypan, continue cooking uncooked portion.

Vegetables

Spiced Zucchini Eggplant

2 zucchini, ends cut, sliced into ¼" discs
1 eggplant, ends cut, sliced into ½" discs
1 red bell pepper, cored, pencil size slices
2 cloves garlic, minced
½ onion, minced
1 cup tomato puree
2 Tbsp olive oil, divided
¼ tsp oregano
Pinch red pepper flakes
Pinch cayenne pepper
Sea salt and pepper to taste

Mix puree, garlic, onion, spices, ½ olive oil in large baking dish.
Place vegetable rings slightly overlapping, alternating vegies.
Drizzle remaining oil on top, cover dish.
Bake @ 375F for one hour.

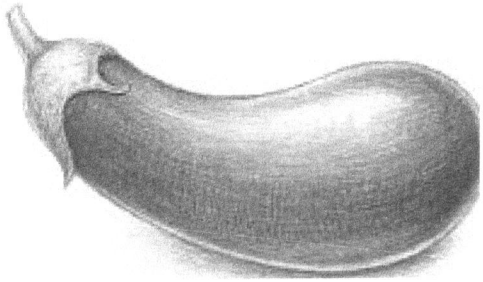

Eggplant Tapas

2 eggplants, large
2 eggs, beaten
1 cup harina
¼ cup parmesan chest
1 Tbsp water
½ tsp sea salt
½ tsp pepper

Eggplant is widely used in Caribbean cooking, especially as roast chips, tapas.

Slice eggplants into ½" discs, salt both sides, drain on screen 30 min.
Mix harina, cheese, spice on dinner plate, spread evenly.
Whisk egg with water, pour on to 2nd plate.
Dry discs, coat in egg, coat on harina, put aside on 3rd plate.
Cover large trays with foil, evenly place discs.
Bake @ 400F for 30 min, turn over and cook 15 min other side.

Baigan Venezolano (eggplant)

1 large eggplant eggplants, cut into large cubes
2 Tbsp olive oil, divided
4 cups onion, sliced
2 cloves garlic, minced
1 tsp sea salt
½ tsp pepper
½ tsp cinnamon
3 tomatoes, coarsely chopped
1 can garbanzo beans, rinsed and drained

Heat large frypan med, sauté eggplant in ½ oil 8 min.
Put eggplant in bowl, set aside.
In same frypan, sauté onions in remaining oil until tender.
Stir in garlic, salt, cinnamon, peppers, then sauté 2 or 3 min.
Fold in eggplant, tomatoes, garbanzos in liquid, bring to boil.
Reduce heat, cover, simmer 30 min until all is tender.
Remove cover, cook 15 min until most liquid is absorbed.

CAREFREE CARIBBEAN WEIGHTLOSS ～ 160

Broccoli Tomato Sauté

2 tomatoes, chopped
1 head broccoli, chopped (can also be done with frozen broccoli)
1 onion, cut into wedges
2 garlic cloves, thinly sliced
1 Tbsp olive oil
1 tsp oregano
Heat frypan to medium, add oil.
Sauté onion several min, then garlic, then broccoli.
Add tomato, sauté all for 6 to 8 min.

Haitian Broccoli

1 large broccoli, cut into small heads
1 medium onion, diced
1 carrot, diced
2 stalks celery, diced
1 Tbsp hot pepper, minced (Jalapeno hot or Anaheim mild)
1 Tbsp coconut oil
Sea salt and pepper to taste
Heat large frypan to medium, add oil.
Sauté onion 3 min.
Add all ingredients, sauté 10 min, stir being careful not to brown it.

Lime Broccoli

1 head broccoli, cut into florets
6 cloves garlic, peeled, smashed
2 lime, zest and juice, divided
¼ cup coconut oil
Pinch sea salt and pepper
¼ cup cilantro, chopped
Mix broccoli, garlic, oil, spices, and ½ lime in large baking dish.
Roast @ 350F for 30 min stirring once.
Sprinkle remaining lime and zest.

Cauliflower Sauté (cauliflower rice)
1 large cauliflower, cut into large pieces
2 Tbsp olive oil
Sea salt and pepper to taste
Use food processor to make cauliflower into rice size pieces.
Heat oil in frypan on medium, add cauliflower.
Cover, stirring occasionally, 5 min, remove from heat.

Roasted Cauliflower with Garlic
1 head cauliflower, cut into 2" florets
6 cloves garlic, peeled and smashed
3 Tbsp olive oil
½ tsp sea salt
¼ tsp oregano
¼ tsp basil
Mix all ingredients in large baking dish.
Bake 1 hour @ 425F, stirring several times.

Roasted Green Beans
1 pound green beans, washed, ends removed.
1 Tbsp olive oil
1 tsp thyme
Sea salt and pepper to taste
Place beans in large glass baking dish.
Sprinkle oil and spices, mix well.
Bake @ 350F for 20 min, tossing occasionally.

Espinacas con Ajo (garlic spinach)
1 bag (appx 10 oz) organic spinach
3 Tbsp pork pieces including drippings
4 garlic cloves, finely minced
1 Tbsp olive oil
1 lime, juiced
½ tsp sea salt
Heat pork and oils at medium in large pot, add garlic, stir 2 min.
Reduce heat, add spinach, salt, pepper stir 3 – 4 min.

Espinacas con Garbanzos

2 cups cooked garbanzo beans
1 bag (appx 10 oz) organic spinach
¼ cup tomato sauce
3 garlic cloves, finely minced
4 Tbsp olive oil, divided
2 Tbsp balsamic vinegar
½ tsp cumin
Sea salt and pepper to taste
Pinch of cayenne pepper

Heat large frypan on medium high, add 1/2 oil.
Sauté spinach briefly until wilted, remove to strain.
Add remaining oil to pan, add garlic, spices, ½ garbanzos, sauté 2 min.
Put sautéed mix into blender, add balsamic vinegar, blend briefly.
Return blended mix to frypan, add remaining garbanzos, tomato sauce.
Cook 5 min, stir occasionally, perhaps add water to slightly thin mix.
Add spinach, gently stir, serve.
Drizzle a little olive oil on top, sprinkle paprika and fresh pepper.

Jamaican Callaloo

1 bunch fresh callaloo kale or collard greens (appx 1 ½ pounds)
3 ripe plantains, peeled, sliced lengthwise medium thick
½ cup leftover pork, cut into small pieces
3 garlic cloves, minced
1 onion, medium, sliced thin
1 tomato, diced
1 Jalapeno or Anaheim pepper
2 Tbsp coconut oil
½ tsp paprika (smoked paprika best)
Sea salt and pepper to taste

Cut leaves from stems, cut in chunks, soak in cold water 5 min.
Oil frypan with thin coat, Sauté pork till crispy, add onions, garlic, thyme.
Add tomatoes, whole pepper, paprika, salt, black pepper, sauté 2 min.
Add greens, cover for 8 min, add a little water as needed to keep steam.
In separate frypan, heat oil on medium, fry plantains turning often.
When plantains are browned, sprinkle with salt and pepper.
Pup hot Callaloo on plate, serve with hot plantains.

Calabacin (zucchini and pepper)

4 small green zucchinis, diced into ½" pieces
1 red bell pepper, sliced pencil sized
1 hot pepper (Jalapeno or Anaheim) cored, seeded, sliced
1 medium onion, minced
3 garlic cloves, minced
3 Tbsp olive oil
2 Tbsp cilantro, chopped
½ tsp oregano
¼ tsp cumin
Sea salt and pepper to taste
¼ cup Parmesan cheese, garnish
Heat frypan to medium, add oil.
Sauté hot pepper, then add onion, cook stirring 5 min.
Add garlic and spices, sauté another 2 min.
Add red bell pepper, zucchini, sauté 6 – 8 min until tender.
Remove from heat, sprinkle on cilantro and Parmesan.

Roast Beets with Carrots

1 large beet, peeled, cut into 1" cubes.
2 medium carrots, peeled, cut into 1" lengths.
3 garlic cloves, thinly sliced
3 Tbsp coconut oil
Sea salt and liberal use of ground pepper
Pinch cayenne pepper
Pinch turmeric
Heat oil in sauce pan on medium, add garlic and spices.
Blend all in glass baking dish with lid, bake @ 425F 15 min.

Balsamic Beets

1 – 2 beets, peeled and cut into 1" cubes
1 Tbsp coconut oil
1 Tbsp balsamic vinegar
½ tsp sea salt.
Preheat oven @ 400F.
Put all ingredients in large glass baking dish.
Roast uncovered 40 minutes, or until tender.

Mexican Street Corn
4 ears corn on cob, corn sliced off from cob
2 cloves garlic, minced
1 lime zested and juiced
2 Tbsp olive oil, divided
1 hot pepper, either hot or mild, cored, diced
1 red bell pepper, cored, diced
1 tomato, medium, diced
½ cup cilantro, finely chopped
½ tsp chili powder
Sea salt and pepper to taste
Heat frypan medium, add ½ olive oil, then add garlic for 2 min.
Add corn, red pepper, 3 min undisturbed, flip over 2 min undisturbed.
Flip over again, add oil, chili, cilantro, lime zest and juice, spices.
Add tomato last, stir, finish cooking 2 – 3 min.

Meat and chicken

Croquetas
2 cups chopped chicken, shellfish, salmon, octopus, or pork
2 eggs, beaten
1 cup leftover boiled yuca, mashed with fork
3 Tbsp coconut oil, divided
¼ cup cilantro, chopped
½ onion, chopped
1 lime, zested, juiced
½ tsp paprika
¼ tsp cayenne
Sea salt and pepper to taste
In large bowl, beat eggs, ½ oil, lime juice and spices.
Mix in meat, onion, cilantro, yuca, chill for 20 min.
Coat bottom of large cooking plate or tray with remaining oil.
Form golf ball sized croquets from cold mixture.
Flatten golf ball size into ½" thick paddies.
Bake @ 400F for 30 – 40 min.

Albondigas (Cuban meat balls)

1 lb. ground beef or pork, blended is best
2 cups tomatoes, crushed (can be canned)
2 Tbsp olive oil, divided
1 onion, minced
2 cloves garlic, minced
1 egg
1 cup leftover boiled yuca, boiled then mashed
½ cup red wine
1 tsp paprika
1 Tbsp fresh cilantro, chopped
1 tsp sea salt
¼ tsp pepper

Heat 2 tsp oil in frypan on medium, sauté ½ onion and garlic 3 min.
In large bowl mix meat, egg, cilantro, salt and pepper.
Add onion mix after it cools, add yuca, mix with hands.
Heat remaining oil, add walnut size balls of hand rolled mix, don't crowd.
Briefly sauté 5 – 7 min, turning to brown all sides, set aside.
Sauté remaining onion 3 min.
Mix in crushed tomatoes, wine, paprika, and salt.
Reduce heat to medium low, add balls, simmer 20 min.

Cuban Pulled Pork

3 – 4 lb. pork roast
4 cloves garlic minced
¾ tsp cumin
2 tsp oregano
1 tsp sea salt
2 Tbsp olive oil, divided
½ cup lime + grapefruit juice, fresh

Mix garlic, cumin, oregano, salt + ½ oil in bowl, massage into pork.
Seal bowl, marinate overnight in refrigerator.
Turn slow-cooker to low, add meat and ½ oil, add marinade.
Cook 8 hours, baste often with juices.
Put meat on plate, shred using forks.

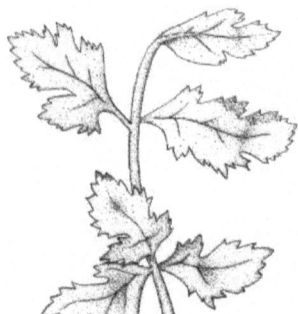

Cilantro is a regular flavor herb used throughout the Caribbean. It is unique because it detoxifies the liver.

Caribbean Harvest Chicken Soup

1 *whole chicken, cut into 4 parts*
½ *gallon water (add more as needed)*
2 *green plantains, cut into 2" pieces*
2 *medium carrots, cut into thick discs*
2 *ears of corn, cut into 2" pieces*
1 *yuca root, peeled cut into 2" pieces*
1 *celery stalk, diced*
½ *squash, butternut, diced*
½ *red bell pepper, seeded, chopped*
½ *green bell pepper, seeded, chopped*
½ *onion, diced*
4 *cloves garlic, diced*
1 *hot pepper, Jalapeno or Anaheim, seeded and diced*
1 *red bell pepper, diced*
2 *Tbsp olive oil*
2 *tsp cumin*
3 *tsp oregano*
1 *tsp sea salt*
1 *cups cilantro, chopped*
Sea salt and pepper to taste

Puree garlic, carrots, peppers, onion, and ½ cilantro.
In large pot combine puree with water, spices.
Bring to boil, then lower heat, simmer 10 min.
Add chicken and spices simmer 30 min.
Add yucca, corn, squash, and plantains, simmer 20 min.
Serve with remaining cilantro sprinkled on.

Ropa Vieja ("old clothes")

2 pounds pork or beef
2 onions, quartered (one for water, other for sauté pan)
1 tomato, quartered
1 carrot, cut into ½" pieces
½ green bell pepper, thinly sliced
½ red bell pepper, thinly sliced
2 garlic cloves, minced
2 Tbsp olive oil
1 tsp cumin
½ cup tomato paste
½ cup wine
Sea salt and pepper to taste

Put 6 cups water in large pot with meat, onion, tomato, carrot, garlic.
Boil, skim off surface oils and foam, then reduce to simmer 45 min.
Remove meat, strain, allow to cool, save broth.
On dinner plate with 2 forks, shred meat into spaghetti sized strips.
Sauté vegetables from the broth, peppers, cook 4 min.
Add meat, spices, puree, wine, sauté 5 min, remove from heat.

Picadillo Cubano (Cuban ground meat)

4 tomatoes, chopped
2 Tbsp balsamic vinegar
1 tsp cinnamon
1 tsp cumin
2 bay leaves
Pinch ground clove
½ tsp sea salt
½ tsp pepper

Heat oil in large frypan at medium, add onions, garlic, stir 5 min.
Add meat, salt, pepper, stir and sauté 5 – 7 min.
Add tomatoes, vinegar, spices, cover pan, reduce heat 30 min.
Remove cover, add raisins, olives, stir and sauté 15 min.

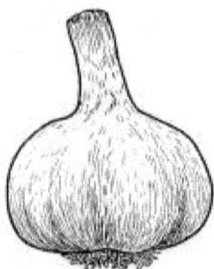

Garlic is very low in toxins and used so often in Caribbean cooking you may want to get a mashing tool or mortar and pestle.

Mexican Tomato Pork Chili
2 – 3 pounds pork or beef
4 tomatoes, chopped
3 peppers (hot or mild) seeded, cut into long strips
3 limes, zested and juiced e
2 cloves garlic, minced
2 Tbsp coconut oil
2 tsp oregano
½ tsp cumin
¼ tsp cayenne pepper
¼ tsp red pepper flakes
Sea salt, pepper to taste
¼ cup cilantro, chopped (for garnish)
Put everything in slow cooker, cook low 8 – 10 hours

Beefsteak Vinaigrette
2 thick steaks, cut into ¼" thick strips
½ onion, diced
2 Tbsp coconut oil
¼ cup sweet balsamic vinegar
½ tsp cayenne pepper
¼ tsp dry mustard
Salt and pepper (generous) to taste
½ sweet red pepper, diced
Marinade all but red pepper at least one hour.
Sauté 8 – 10min in med heat frypan, add red pepper last minutes.
Serve sprinkled with fresh cilantro.

Caribbean Seafood

Caribbean Ceviche
1 – 2 lbs. mixed shellfish
2 cups lime juice
½ red onion, sliced razor thin
1 cup tomatoes, seeded, sliced thin
½ cup hot pepper, Jalapeno (hot) or Anaheim (mild)
2 tsp sea salt
Pinch oregano
Pinch cayenne pepper
1 Tbsp cilantro, chopped
Put unfrozen shellfish in bowl, rinse, dry with towel.
Mix all ingredients in bowl, let chill one hour

Caribbean Paella
1 – 2 lbs. shellfish, thawed, rinsed, dried on paper towel
1 onion, chopped
2 cloves garlic, chopped
1 cup long grain rice
1 cup tomatoes, diced
1 cup frozen green peas, thawed
½ cup green bell peppers, sliced thin
2 Tbsp olive oil
2 cups broth
1 tsp paprika
½ tsp sea salt
¼ tsp pepper
Pinch saffron
Zest of lime
Put 1 cup water in saucepan, cover, boil, lower heat to med.
Add shellfish, cook 4 min, then add onion, garlic cook for 4 min.
Add spices, tomato, broth, bring all to boil, add rice evenly.
Cover, cook on medium 25 min until rice is tender.
Stir in remaining ingredients, cook another 10 min.

Salmon con Tomati

4 large salmon fillets
4 cloves garlic, minced, divided
1 yuca, diced
1 onion, diced
1 can 14 oz roasted diced tomatoes
1 cup tomato sauce
10 stuffed Spanish olives
2 Tbsp olive oil, divided
½ cup broth
1 tsp vinegar
1 bay leaf
½ tsp sea salt
½ tsp pepper
¼ tsp cayenne

Mix ½ garlic, pepper, salt, vinegar, ½ oil.
Use half this to season the fish, set aside.
Heat frypan medium low, add ½ oil.
Sauté onions and ½ garlic 4 minutes, avoid burning.
Add remaining ingredients but not the salmon, cover, cook 15 min.
When yuca is cooked, add salmon, water if needed.
Sauté salmon briefly, 3 min each side at most.

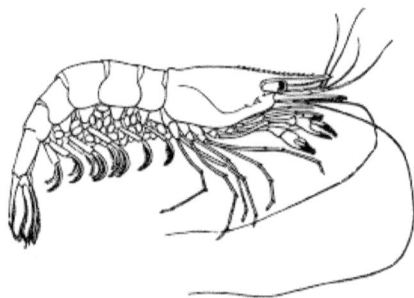

Shellfish are very commonly prepared in Caribbean dishes. Shrimp joins with octopus, squid, muscles, and many small fish such as sardines.

Mariscos de Ron (shellfish in rum sauce)

1 pound mixed shellfish (can be frozen bag)
½ green bell pepper, minced
4 cloves garlic, minced
½ onion, minced
1 cup water, use as needed to sauté vegetables
¼ cup rum
2 Tbsp butter
1 Tbsp olive oil
¼ tsp pepper
¼ tsp cayenne pepper
¼ cup cilantro, chopped
½ tsp sea salt, divided
1 lime, zest and juice (for garnish)

Heat oil in frypan to medium, sauté onion and bell pepper 2 min.
Add spices, ½ salt, reduce heat until thickens, set aside.
Rinse shellfish in cool water, dry on towel, sprinkle with ½ salt.
Heat butter in separate frypan to medium, add garlic, sauté till tender.
Add shellfish, sauté 2 min, add rum and cilantro, sauté 2 min.
Mix with vegetables, serve immediately, sprinkle lime zest and juice.

Mariscos Morrocoy (Venezuelan shellfish)

1 pound mixed shellfish (can be frozen bag)
1 lime, zested and juiced
4 Tbsp coconut oil
2 cloves garlic, minced
2 tsp cilantro, chopped
1 Tbsp paprika
1 tsp sea salt, divided
½ tsp red pepper flakes

Rinse shellfish in cool water, dry on towel sprinkle with ½ salt.
In large bowl, hand mix seafood, oil, garlic, spices.
Heat sauté pan 2 min med high, add mixture.
Sauté and stir 4 minutes, until just opaque, not any longer.
Serve over rice with pan sauces, lime, and sprinkled cilantro.

Gambas al Ajillo (garlic shrimp)

1 – 2 pounds shrimp, shelled and deveined, tails intact
6 cloves garlic, thinly sliced
1/4 cup olive oil
1 hot pepper, Jalapeno (hot) or Anaheim (mild)
½ cup cilantro, chopped
2 Tbsp dry white wine, or whatever you have
2 limes, zested then juiced
½ tsp paprika
Sea salt and pepper to taste
Toasted flatbread for serving

Sauté garlic in oil briefly on medium high.
Add shrimp, peppers, spices, sauté 3 min.
Stir in wine, lime juice, zest, spoon of water, cilantro for 1 min.
Serve immediately, discard pepper.

Bahameil Fish Escabeche (Bahama fish appetizer)

1 pound fish fillets (salmon, haddock, flounder, Atlantic mackerel)
1 cup hernia (cornmeal)
1 green bell pepper, cut in pencil strips
1 red bell pepper, cut in pencil strips
1 onion, cut in pencil strips
1 carrot, cut in pencil strips
1 hot pepper, either hot or mild, seeded, minced
1 cup olive oil, divided
1 cup white vinegar
1 bay leaf
½ tsp sea salt
½ tsp pepper
¼ tsp allspice

Sauté all peppers, onion, carrot in ½ the olive oil.
Stir in vinegar, set all aside in bowl with top.
Season fish with salt and pepper, then dredge in hernia.
Heat frypan again with remaining oil until oil is hot.
Briefly cook fish 2 minutes each side, until half-cooked.
Add to vegetable mix in glassware and cover.
Refrigerate overnight to allow vinegar to finish the cooking.

Trini Shrimp with Rum

2 - 4 pounds large shrimp, deveined with shells on
1 medium tomato, cut into wedges
1 green bell pepper, cut pencil size strips
1 small onion, cut pencil size strips
1 lime zested and juiced
3 Tbsp tomato sauce (mild salsa works great)
¼ cup dark rum
2 tsp soy sauce
¼ tsp ground pepper
2 Tbsp coconut oil
2 cloves garlic, minced
¼ tsp dried ginger
½ tsp sea salt
2 Tbsp cilantro, chopped

In bowl, wash shrimp in lime juice very briefly, then rinse and dry.
In another bowl, mix tomato sauce, rum, soy sauce and pepper.
Heat large frypan on high. Add oil, garlic, ginger, stir 10 sec.
Move garlic to side, add shrimp uncrowded 1 min, undisturbed.
Add salt, mix 30 seconds until shrimp turn orange.
Add tomatoes, peppers, onions, stir fry 1 min.
Add tomato sauce mixture, stir fry 1 min. Stir in cilantro.

Bacalao Dominicana (Dominican cod)

2 lbs. salted dried codfish
2 cups yuca chunks
4 tomatoes, quartered
2 green bell peppers, diced
2 cloves garlic, crushed
1 cup tomato sauce
1 onion, sliced
½ gallon water (plus a cup)
2 Tbsp olive oil
½ cup seeded olives, sliced
¼ cup cilantro, chopped
1 tsp sea salt
½ tsp pepper

Soak cod overnight in water.
Boil yuca until tender, set aside, then boil cod for 8 min.
Remove cod, flake fish, reserve liquid.
In pot on medium heat, add oil, sauté all vegetables until translucent.
Add cup water, simmer low for 3 min. Add codfish, tomato sauce, stir.
Add yuca, salt, pepper, simmer 10 min.

Starches

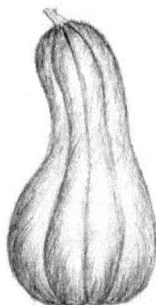

Squash was the first starch used in Mesoamerica and is widely used today. It replaces many potato items as a very healthful vegetable without any of the problems of white potato.

Roasted Squash with Lime
1 large winter squash, cut lengthwise in half
3 Tbsp coconut oil
2 limes, juiced
1 Tbsp honey
1 tsp sea salt
½ tsp pepper
¼ to ½ tsp cayenne pepper, to taste
Remove squash seeds, peel, cut into 1" cubes, mix all ingredients.
Place on cooking pan with space between each.
Roast @ 400F 40 min, turning once.

Mangu
2 plantains
4 Tbsp olive oil
1 tsp sea salt
1 cup warm water

Peel plantains, cut lengthwise into 4 long strips.
Boil water with salt, add plantains, boil until tender.
Remove plantains, put in mixing bowl, fully mash with fork.
Add olive oil on top.

Dedos de Bruja (witches fingers)
1 large winter squash, cut lengthwise in half
2 Tbsp coconut oil
½ tsp sea salt
½ tsp pepper
½ tsp paprika
¼ tsp cayenne pepper
Cut squash into long strips, 4 strips per side.
In bowl, blend oil, spices, and strips of squash, one at a time.
Place coated strips on cooking pan, well-spaced.
Roast @ 400F 40 min, turning once.

Batata Naranja (sweet potato and orange)
4 sweet potatoes
3 oranges, zested and juiced, include some pulp
¼ cup honey
1 coconut oil
½ tsp nutmeg
½ tsp cinnamon
Boil potatoes until barely tender enough to pierce with fork.
Remove from pan, put in bowl of cool water, peel potatoes.
Cut in half lengthwise, place in large shallow baking pan.
Mix remaining ingredients in saucepan, boil, then simmer 2 min.
Pour saucepan ingredients over potatoes.
Bake @ 350F for one hour, baste often until well glazed.

Boiled Yuca
2 medium yuca roots, peeled (can use frozen)
1 lime
1 tsp olive oil
½ tsp sea salt
Boil yuca in large pot of water 20 min or until fork can penetrate.

Roasted Yuca

2 medium yuca roots, peeled (can use frozen)
2 limes, zested, juiced
1 Tbsp olive oil
½ tsp oregano
½ tsp garlic powder
½ tsp cumin
½ tsp sea salt
½ tsp pepper

Boil yuca 15 min, drain, break into 4 chunks, set aside.
In bowl, combine oil, spices, then drench yucca in mix.
Arrange yuca on oiled baking dish or two.
Bake @ 400F for 40 min, or until brown.
Sprinkle with lime juice, serve.

Sautéed Yuca

2 yuca roots, peeled (can use frozen)
2 Tbsp olive oil, divided
½ tsp sea salt

Boil 15 min, drain, cool, cut into long finger sized strips.
On dinner plate, combine ½ oil, spices, then drench yuca in mix.
Heat frypan to medium with oil, sauté 15 min, turning regularly.

Bell peppers of all colors are a regular ingredient. Be sure to always get organic peppers.

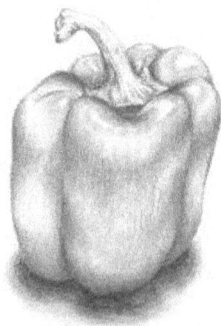

Sweet Potato Purée

2 sweet potatoes
1 Tbsp olive oil
Sea salt and pepper to taste

Boil potatoes until soft.
Remove from pan, put in bowl of cool water, peel potatoes.
In large bowl, mash potatoes briefly with fork.
Add remaining ingredients, make puree with electric beater.

Sweet Potato Crisps
2 – 4 sweet potatoes
1 – 2 Tbsp coconut oil
½ tsp sea salt
½ tsp pepper
1 / 2 tsp paprika
Peel potatoes, cut into "poker chip" disks.
Mix oil and spices in bowl, add potatoes, drench both sides.
Bake on oiled baking sheets @ 425F for 30 min, stirring twice.
Or barbeque 20 min, turning often.

Patacones (tostones)
3 – 4 green plantains
½ cup coconut oil
Sea salt to taste
Peel plantains with knife, cut into 2" round pieces.
Boil in large pot of water 15 - 20 min.
When very hot, press into ½" disks on cutting board.
(Press oiled bottom of a pot on top of boiled plantain to flatten.)
Heat oil in large frypan to medium high, fry each 3 min per side.
Cool and drain on plate with paper towel.

Garbanzos Guisados (garbanzo stew)
1 cup leftover pork, cubed
4 cups cooked garbanzo beans (about 15 oz.)
1 can diced tomatoes with sauce, 28 oz.
1 onion, diced
2 cloves garlic, mashed
1 Tbsp olive oil
¼ cup cilantro, chopped
Pinch red pepper flakes
Sea salt and pepper to taste
Heat olive oil in frypan to medium, add onion, garlic, spices.
Sauté 5 – 7 min stirring often, stir in leftover pork.
Add garbanzos, diced tomatoes, simmer to reduce liquid.
Serve with cilantro sprinkled on top.

Liberally use herbs and spices to bring out the flavor for Caribbean cooking. Regularly build up your spice cabinet as you adapt to new herbs and their combinations.

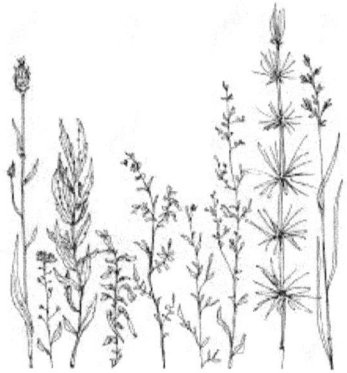

Slow Cooked Beans

3 cups dried beans
1 large onion, finely chopped
1 ½ cup tomato puree
¼ cup tomato paste
1 ½ cups water
½ cup honey
1 Tbsp baking soda
1 Tbsp dry mustard
2 tsp sea salt
½ tsp pepper

In large mixing bowl, cover beans with water and baking soda overnight.
Drain beans, rinse, and rinse again.
Add all to slow cooker, cook on low 8 to 10 hours.

Quinoa Fria (cold quinoa)

½ cup quinoa, washed
½ onion, chopped fine
1 tomato, chopped
1 lime, zested and juiced
½ green bell pepper, chopped
¼ cup cilantro, chopped
Sea salt and pepper to taste

Bring 1 cup water to boil, reduce heat, add quinoa, cover.
When all water is absorbed, remove from heat, mix in all ingredients.
Refrigerate.

Soup and salad

Gazpacho (cold tomato soup)
4 tomatoes
3 cups tomato sauce or puree
3 cloves garlic, minced
2 red bell peppers, cored
1 cucumber, halved, seeded, not peeled
½ cup wine
1 Tbsp pepper
2 tsp sea salt
Dice cucumbers, peppers, tomatoes and onions.
Briefly pulse in blender, careful not to do too much.
Combine all ingredients in large bowl, chill, serve cold.

Sopa de Verduras (vegetable soup)
1 qt cold water
1 cup broth
1 onion, chopped
1 zucchini, chopped
1 celery stalk, chopped with leaves
2 carrots, sliced in thin discs
½ cabbage, core removed, chopped
1 cup green string beans, cut 1"
1 cup peas (frozen, add just before serving)
1 cup garbanzo beans, soaked overnight, rinsed
1 cup black beans, soaked overnight, rinsed
8 oz can tomato paste
½ cup rice
¼ cup cilantro, chopped
¼ tsp cumin
Sea salt, pepper to taste
Place all ingredients in slow cooker, cook 8 – 10 hours on low.

Salads

Cucumber Salad
4 cucumbers, peeled, cut into discs
¼ onion, sliced very thin
½ cup white vinegar
½ cup water
¼ cup honey
1 tsp dill, or to taste
½ tsp dry mustard
Slice cucumbers into bowl.
Combine other ingredients (but not dill) into saucepan.
Heat, then add dill, then pour over cucumbers, cool one hour.

Avocado Salad Dressing
1 avocado, large, skin removed
½ lemon or lime, juiced
1 clove garlic, crushed
¼ cup water
2 tsp olive oil
1 tsp dill
1 tsp honey
½ tsp sea salt
Place all ingredients in bowl, blend with fork, then whisk until fluffy.
Cool in refrigerator one hour.

Ensalada Puertoriquena
3 tomatoes, chopped
2 avocados, chopped
1 cucumber, peeled and sliced
1 Anaheim or mild pepper, seeded, chopped
½ onion, sliced paper thin
1 lime, juiced
2 Tbsp olive oil
Salt, pepper to taste
Toss and serve with flatbread

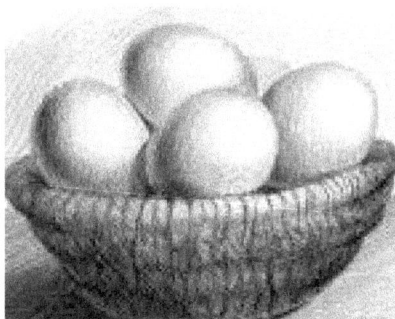

Cesar Salad Dressing

1 egg yolk, room temperature
½ cup mild olive oil, divided
3 limes, juiced
1 Tbsp dijon mustard
¼ cup parmesan cheese, grated
¼ clove garlic, peeled and crushed
½ tsp sea salt
½ tsp pepper
Pinch cayenne pepper

Have whole fresh eggs daily, mostly due to the fat value from the yolks.

Add egg yolks, garlic, lime juice, dijon to blender, pulse 5 times.
Remove plug from lid, turn blender on low and slowly drizzle ½ oil.
Turn blender off, add salt, pepper, cayenne.
Turn blender on, slowly drizzle remaining oil.
Turn blender off, add parmesan, pulse 5 times.

Ensalada de Repollo (coleslaw)

1 cabbage head, shredded thin
1 red bell pepper, sliced thin
½ onion, sliced thin
3 carrots, peeled, shredded thin
3 limes, zested and juiced
½ cup olive oil
½ cup cilantro, chopped thin
¼ cup honey
¼ cup sweet balsamic vinegar
½ tsp cumin
¼ tsp cayenne pepper
Sea salt and pepper to taste

Blend all in large bowl, chill in refrigerator 2 hours.

Caribbean Cocktails (*Tragos Caribe*)

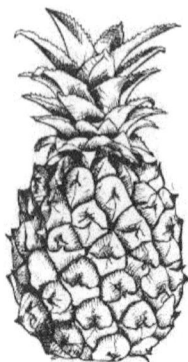

The best Pina Coladas are made with fresh pineapple in food processor, blended to a pulp, then the juice strained including some pulp. Then do same with coconut.

Pina Colada
2 cups fresh pineapple, peeled, blended into pulp, strained
2 oz coconut milk, unsweetened, or fresh strained from food processor
4 oz rum (white rum is lighter taste)
2 Tbsp honey, ice
Blend pineapple, rum, honey, coconut milk, ice until smooth.
Serve over ice in large glasses with flair.

Sangria Caribe
1 apple, cored, diced
1 lime, sliced thin
½ cup pineapple, diced
1 orange, seeded, sliced thin
2 oranges, juiced
2 Tbsp honey
½ - 1 cup rum
1 or 2 bottles (25 oz ea.) red wine
Club soda, chilled
In large pitcher, stir apples, oranges, juice.
Stir in wine, rum, orange juice, honey until well mixed.
Refrigerate 4 hours or overnight.
Pour over ice in glass, top with soda, stir.

Mojito

2 oz rum
½ lime squeezed
1 tsp honey (dissolved in a little water)
3 mint leaves
Club soda to taste
In cocktail glass, mash lime juice with sugar.
Add mint leaves, mashing them to bottom of glass.
Fill glass 2/3 with cracked ice, add rum, soda, mix by hand.

Margarita Carefree

2 oz tequila
2 oz water
1 tsp honey (dissolved in the little water)
1 ½ oz lime juice, fresh squeezed
½ oz orange juice, fresh squeezed
In jar with top, add lime, orange, water, tequila, honey mix, stir.
Add ice, cover top and shake.
Holding cocktail glass upside down, dip rim into salt.
Add Margarita to glass.

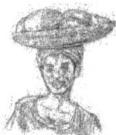

Ten

LAST DANCE

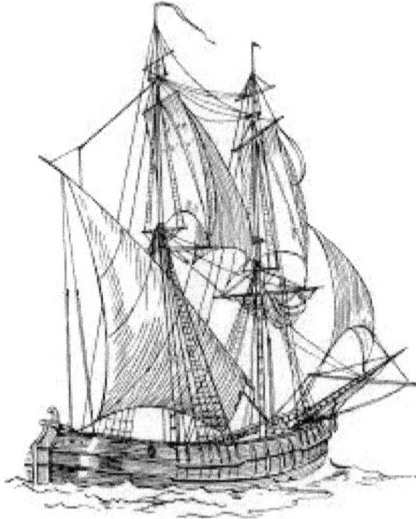

"The real voyage of discovery consists not in seeking new landscapes,
but in having new eyes."
~ Marcel Proust

Don't make this change expensive. Don't make it a list of rules you absolutely must follow or else. Don't overthink it to the point where you become robotic. Stop all negative thoughts and all self-doubt, especially that voice in the back of your mind that says you can't succeed.

Instead, imagine what being successful will be like. Think about how much money you're going to save. This should save you several thousand dollars over the next few years in money that won't be wasted. There are things you need to get started, and things you'll need to get along the way. However, there's no need to rush to buy exotic items, no need to go hunting for tiny stores in the middle of nowhere. You need to have kitchen essentials to cook and store food, but absolutely not equipping yourself for Top Chef competition.

Much of what you have now will do the job, but you'll definitely need to cook in cast iron or glass. Stainless steel will be safe if it is quite high quality because the lower the quality, the cheaper metal fillers, most typically nickel which can flake off. It's a good idea to get a big cast iron or ceramic pot for cooking the many soup and stew dishes you'll have. Be sure to have lids for cooking along with wooden spatulas and stir spoons.

You can buy clean, mostly organic food at your grocery store. Latin food ingredients that make up most of the meals you'll prepare are widely available, but some of the specialty items may need to be ordered online from Amazon or other sources. By following the lists provided here, you'll easily remove 80% of the toxins that are typical in food and households.

Grocery stores usually offer cage free chicken, cage free eggs, organic butter, and organic Greek Yogurt. Overall, milk products should be consumed at a minimum due to the high rate of toxins and the high amount of milk sugar. However, if you can get feta cheese (made from sheep and goat's milk) try to get some into your meals, often sprinkled on salads. The health value is tremendous, the fats feature a large percentage of omega-3, feta cheese has very high amounts of vitamins and minerals, and the processing uses very low amount of preservatives. You'll find feta cheese at many grocery stores and at a large organic store.

It's easy to get good quality meat at your grocery store and health food stores. At the grocery store grass fed beef, pork, and even bison will usually be offered at prices not much higher than non-grass fed.

A third option provides super quality meats at affordable prices; however you need to buy in bulk. You can order frozen grass fed meat from Amazon, shipped straight from the ranch. A much better choice is *EatWild.com*, which has an expansive list of 1,400 ranches reasonably close to you that ship meat and dairy directly to you. To get the experience of it all, try to drive to a ranch, enjoy the scenery, and buy directly.

Buying seafood is more problematic. Your grocery store doesn't categorize fish into those with the highest mercury or contaminant levels, and frozen fish tends to come from fish farms in China. "Fish markets" are hard to find for most people, and what is sold can be a toxic nightmare. However, with an EWG list of fish lowest in contaminants and where to find them, you don't need to wander about hunting for fish markets.

Frozen Wild Alaskan Salmon is easy to find in most grocery stores, along with frozen Pacific cod, Alaskan pollock, and haddock. Grocery stores with a larger selection of fresh fish will often have frozen fish that maintains quality longer, is easy to prepare, and easily fits into busy lifestyle. The fish are quickly frozen within hours of harvest so they are quite fresh.

Caribbean fishermen find shellfish near the shore, often with labor intensive work getting them from rocky areas and hard to find cervices. Due to this difficulty, these shellfish are sold all over the Caribbean in the tiny harbor fish markets. Crab and lobster obviously go to the restaurants to serve to tourists, so the locals get a great selection of local shellfish along with squid, octopus, and sardines. The same goes for those of us up north. Great frozen shellfish bags can easily be purchased at local grocery stores at surprisingly affordable prices.

Shopping for the essentials

Vegetables:	*Doesn't need to be organic*		*Should be organic*
Asparagus	✓		
Avocado	✓		
Beets		50/50	
Bell peppers (all colors)			✓
Broccoli	✓		
Cabbage	✓		
Carrots			✓
Cauliflower	✓		
Celery			✓
Cilantro			✓
Cucumber			✓
Eggplant	✓		

	Doesn't need to be organic	Should be organic
Garlic	✓	
Green beans (string beans)		✓
Kale		✓
Lettuce (Romaine)		✓
Mushrooms	✓	
Onions	✓	
Peas, (sweet)	✓	
Peppers (hot)		✓
Spinach		✓
Sweet corn	✓	
Tomatoes		✓
Zucchini	✓	

Fruit:	*Doesn't need to be organic*	*Should be organic*
Blueberries, blackberries		✓
Coconut	✓	
Grapefruit	✓	
Lemons		✓
Limes		✓
Oranges		✓
Pineapple	✓	
Papaya	✓	

Starches:	*Doesn't need to be organic*	*Should be organic*
Plantains	✓	
Quinoa	✓	
Rice	✓	
Squash, winter	50/50	
Sweet potato	✓	
White potato (Russet)		✓
Yuca	✓	

Legumes:	*Doesn't need to be organic*	*Should be organic*
Garbanzo beans	✓	
Lentils	✓	
Navy beans	✓	
Red beans	✓	

Nuts and seeds:	Doesn't need to be organic	Should be organic
Almonds		✓
Brazil nuts		✓
Cashews		✓
Pumpkin seeds	✓	
Walnuts	50/50	

Protein:	Doesn't need to be free range	Should be free range
Beef		✓
Bison		✓
Dairy (Greek yogurt, hard cheese)		✓
Eggs		✓
Pork		✓
Poultry		✓

Seafood:	Doesn't need to be special	Should be special
Anchovies	✓	
Atlantic mackerel	✓	
Cod	✓	
Pollock	✓	
Haddock	✓	
Halibut (Pacific)		✓
Herring	✓	
Muscles	✓	
Octopus (Pacific)		✓
Oysters	✓	
Rainbow trout (should come from cold lakes)		✓
Salmon (must state "Wild Alaskan Salmon")		✓
Shrimp (should come from West Coast US)		✓
Squid	✓	

*Frozen produce rated excellent, canned often problematic due to chemical treatment.
**Hothouse produce is generally grown without chemicals fertilizers or pesticides.
***Canned or frozen fish – read label carefully to avoid chemical additives.

Spices:	Doesn't need to be organic	Should be organic
Basil	✓	
Bay leaves	✓	
Black peppercorns	✓	
Cayenne pepper	✓	
Cinnamon	✓	
Cumin	✓	
Mustard, ground	✓	
Oregano	✓	
Paprika	✓	
Saffron	✓	
Sea salt	✓	
Thyme	✓	
Turmeric	✓	

Specialty essentials	If you can't find it try
Cassava flour	Amazon
Curtido (Salvadorian sauerkraut)	Amazon
Fish oil or fish oil capsules	Amazon
Garbanzo flour	Amazon
Green tea, loose leaf	Amazon
Pickled beets (organic)	Amazon
Wild honey	Amazon

Kitchen essentials	If you can't find it try
Iron fry pans	Walmart, Amazon
Stainless steel pots and pans	Walmart, Amazon
Glass, ceramic cookware	Walmart, Amazon
Glass storage jars	Walmart, Amazon
Slow cooker (crock pot)	Walmart, Amazon
Citrus zester	Amazon
Vegetable choppers	Walmart, Amazon
Wooden spoons, spatulas	Walmart, Amazon

Balance exercise accessories	
Tennis balls	Walmart, Amazon
Playground balls	Walmart, Amazon

Jump ropes	Walmart, Amazon
Medicine balls	Walmart, Amazon
Bulgarian bag components (duffel bag, sand)	Walmart, Amazon
Dumbbells	Walmart
Milk crates	Walmart
Suspension cords (TRX)	Walmart, Amazon

Supplements

"The supplement business is a cruel and shallow money trench, a long plastic hallway where thieves and pimps run free, and good men die like dogs. There's also a negative side."
~ Hunter S. Thompson

Avoid supplements whenever you can. Buy fresh food, cook it yourself. This is what grandmother did and where nutrients should come from.

YouTube Caribbean and Latin cooking

Caribbean Pot (Trinidad and all Caribbean oriented)
Chef Ricardo Cooking (Jamaica, via London)
EcoRico TV (Puerto Rican oriented)
You Can Cook (Venezuelan oriented)
Chef Zee Cooks (Dominican oriented)
How To Cook Mexican Food (Mexican oriented)

Some YouTube attitude adjustment

Get Happy Volkswagen
Malibu Rum Traffic Jam in Jamaica
A Guide to Cuban Coffee
Getting Lost in Guadeloupe
Americans Try Haitian Food First Time
Latinos Try Venezuelan Hallacas
People Try Salvadoran Food
People Taste Test Puerto Rican Food
When Gringos Can't Dance Call The Latin Dance Specialist

Required music

"Without music, life would be a mistake."

~ Friedrich Nietzsche

Latin music is essential. Please, no excuses, just go with the flow. This entire Carefree system is built around the culture of the Islands, and the music is part of Caribbean blood. The goal of this weightloss system is for you to be successful for four years so that you become one of the few percentage of people who beat the odds. It will take a unique attitude, and Latin music will be of tremendous help to put you into the right mindset.

A few of the recommend songs are in English, a few bi-lingual, most are in Spanish. Your job is to feel it, to hum along with it, to let your heart sing. Don't listen like a music critic, listen to find a new way to have fun. Listen all the way through each offering several times, then mark your favorites. When you find a particular artist you like, look up more of their songs.

Find most on YouTube so you can see the dancing, connect with the singer, dive into their story. For example, start with the salsa music of Mandinga. This is a great band featuring a singer from Spain leading a fascinating international ensemble, including musicians from Romania. The songs are mostly in English, but you're guaranteed to feel the salsa sound. Watch Lucy Grau, Leslie Grace, Romeo Santos in great bilingual Latin songs. Watch some eye popping Caribbean dancing to amazing music, especially Marka Registrada in Havana.

Set up your play list of favorites, but here is a start. Time for some energy!

Mandinga, *Hello*	English
Mandinga, *We Don't Talk*	English
Mandinga, *Arquitectura*	Spanish, great salsa dancing
Lucy Grau, *Last Dance*	English/Spanish
Leslie Grace, *Be My Baby*	English/Spanish
Leslie Grace, *Will You Still Love Me*	English/Spanish
Leslie Grace, *Como Duele*	Spanish

Romeo Santos, *Promise*	English/Spanish
Romeo Santos, *Solo Por Un Beso Dance*	Spanish, great bachata dancing
Katanah, *Wrecking Ball*	Spanish/English
Marka Registrada, *Perdoname*	Spanish, great salsa dancing
El Dany, *Te Espere*	Spanish, great salsa dancing
Los Jefes, *Yo Te Prometo*	Spanish, great salsa dancing
Marc Anthony, *Valio La Pena*	Spanish, salsa
Marc Anthony, *Vivir Mi Vida*	Spanish, salsa
Marc Anthony y Natalia, *Recuerdame*	Spanish
Hector Acosta, *Aprendere*	Spanish, bachata
Hector Acosta, *Me Duele*	Spanish, bachata
Hector Acosta, *No Soy un Hombre*	Spanish, bachata
Monchy y Alexandra, *Dos Locos*	Spanish, bachata
Monchy y Alexandra, *Hoja En Blanco*	Spanish, bachata
Xtreme, *Te Extrano*	Spanish, bachata
Havana Lounge de Cuba, *Campina*	Spanish, salsa
Grupo Niche, *Sin Sentimiento*	Spanish, salsa
Grupo Niche, *Cali*	Spanish, salsa
Willy Chirino, *Soy Guajiro*	Spanish, salsa
Rey Ruiz, *Creo En El Amor*	Spanish, salsa
Matias Damasio, *Loucos*	Portuguese, Caribbean
Chino y Nacho, *Me Voy Enamorando*	Spanish, contemporary
Elvis Crespo, *Suavemente*	Spanish, Dominican
Olga Tanon, *Desilucioname*	Spanish, Puerto Rican passion
Gilberto Santa Rosa, *Vivir Sin Ella*	Spanish
Gente de Zona, *La Gozadera*	Spanish
Gente de Zona, *Si No Vuelves*	Spanish
Ozuna, *Dile Que Tu Me Quieres*	Spanish

Statements that are sure ways to fail

"But I'm not from the Caribbean."
"I'm a picky eater."
"I don't like that."
"I can't do that"
"That's not my way"
"I hate…"

Science writers to follow

Dr. Mary Enig
Dr. Robert Lustig
Dr. William Davis
Dr. Pamela Peeke
Dr. Mark Hyman
Dr. Joseph Mercola
Dr. Stephanie Seneff
Dr. Paula Baille-Hamilton
Dr. Bruce Blumberg
Dr. Eric Berg
Michael Pollan
Gary Taubes
Mark Sisson

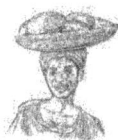

NOTES

Chapter 1

1. Sartorelli, D., et al. High intake of fruits and vegetables predicts weight loss in Brazilian overweight adults. *Nutrition Research Journal*, April 2008.
2. Secor, E., et al. Bromelain inhibits allergic sensitization and murine asthma via modulation of dendritic cells. *Evidence Based Complementary Alternative Medicine*, December 2013.
3. Prior, A., et al. Cholesterol, coconuts and diet on Polynesian atolls. *American Journal of Clinical Nutrition*, 1981.
4. Peeke, P., *Body for Life for Women: A Woman's Plan for Physical and Mental Transformation*. Rodale Books 2009.
5. Wilson, J. Adrenal Fatigue: The 21st Century Stress Syndrome. *Smart Publications,* 2001.
6. Mozaffarian, D., et al. Changes in diet and lifestyle and long-term weight gain in women and men. *New England Journal of Medicine*, June 2011.
7. Grun, F., and Blumberg, B. Minireview: The case for obesogens. *Molecular Endocrinology*, August 2009.
8. Wang, S., et al, Resveratrol induces brown-like adipocyte formation in white fat through activation of AMP-activated protein kinase (AMPK) a1". *International Journal of Obesity*, October 2015.
9. Westererp-Plantenga, M., et al. Metabolic effects of spices, teas, and caffeine. *Physiology and Behavior*, August 2006.
10. Harvie, M., et al. The effects of intermittent or continuous energy restriction on weight loss and metabolic risk disease markers: A randomized trial in young   overweight women. *International Journal of Obesity*, May 2010.
11. Wu, A., et al. Tea and circulating estrogen levels in postmenopausal Chinese women in Singapore. *Oxford Journals, Molecular Carcinogenesis,* May 2005.

Chapter 2

1. Mann, T., et al. Medicare's search for effective obesity treatments: diets are not the answer. *American Psychologist*, April 2007.
2. _____. Global weight loss and gain market (2009 – 2014). *Marketsandmarkets.com.*, accessed February 2018.
3. _____. Obesity and overweight fast starts. Centers for Disease Control and Prevention, *cdc.gov/nchs.*, accessed February 2018.
4. Pietilainen, K., et al. Does dieting make you fat? A twin study. *International Journal of Obesity*, March 2012.
5. Wilson, J., et al. Concurrent training: A meta analysis examining interference of aerobic and resistance exercise. *Journal of Strength and Conditioning Research*, August 2012.
6. Sawyer, BJ., et al. Predictors of fat mass changes in response to aerobic exercise training in women. *Journal of Strength and Conditioning Research*, February 2015.
7. Lally, P., et al. How are habits formed: Modeling habit formation in the real world. *European Journal of Social Psychology*, July 2009.
8. Lally, P., et al. Making health habitual: The psychology of 'habit-formation' and general practice. *The British Journal of General Practice*, December 2012.
9. Marquart, M. Defective joy gene: Study finds Germans incapable of enjoying life. *Spiegel Online International*, May 2012.
10. Marquart, Ibid.

Chapter 3

1. Bienerstock, J., et al. Ingestion of Lactobacillus strain regulates emotional behavior and central GABA receptor expression in a mouse via the vagus nerve. *Proceedings of the National Academy of Sciences.* July 2011.
2. Rind, R. Addressing thyroid and adrenal insufficiency. *Weston A. Price Foundation*, June 2009.
3. _____. Abdominal fat and what to do about it. Harvard Medical School, *Harvard Health Publications*, October 2015.

4. Stenblom, EL., et al, Consumption of thylakoid-rich spinach extract reduces hunger, increases satiety and reduces cravings for palatable food in overweight women. *Elsevier*, August 2015.

5. Streeter, C., et al. Effects of yoga versus walking on mood, anxiety, and brain GABA levels: A randomized controlled MRS study. *Journal of Alternative and Complementary Medicine*, November 2010.

6. Mozaffarian, D., MD et al, Changes in diet and lifestyle and long-term weight gain in women and men, *New England Journal of Medicine*, June 2011.

7. Surninski, R., et al. Acute effect of amino acid ingestion and resistance exercise on plasma growth hormone concentration in young me. *International Journal of Sport Nutrition*, July 1997.

8. Blanchette, K. *Prevention of the Disease of Aging*. Xulon Press, 2007.

9. Wang, C, and Liao, J. A mouse model of diet-induced obesity and insulin resistance. Methods in Molecular Biology, *Springer Science Media*, 2012.

10. Russell, WR, et al. High-protein, reduced-carbohydrate weight-loss diets promote metabolite profiles likely to be detrimental to colonic health. *American Journal of Clinical Nutrition*, May 2011.

11. Saad, F., et al. Testosterone as potential effective therapy in treatment of obesity in men with testosterone deficiency: A review. *Current Diabetes Reviews*, March 2012.

12. Wang, C., et al. Low-fat high-fiber diet decreased serum and urine androgens in men. *Journal of Clinical Endocrinology and Metabolism*. June 2005.

13. MacKelvie, K., et al. Bone mineral density and serum testosterone in chronically trained, high mileage 40-55 year old male runners. *British Journal of Sports Medicine*, August 2000.

14. Morgentaler, A. Harvard expert shares his thoughts on testosterone-replacement therapy. Harvard Medical School, *Harvard Health Publications*, February 2011.

15. Fung, J. The role of fibre I-hormone obesity. *Intensive Dietary Management*, May 2014.

16. Gottfried, S. 10 Surprising facts about how hormones disrupt your health and weight. *Dr. Sara Gottfried.com.*, accessed December 2017.
17. Jin Noh, H., et al. The relationship between hippocampal volume and cognition in patients with chronic primary insomnia. *Journal of Clinical Neurology*, June 2012.
18. Young, E. The dark side of oxytocin, much more than just a "love hormone." *Discover Science*, November 2010.
19. Sahelian, R. Oxytocin natural ways to increase; benefits and side effects. *Dr. Ray Sabelian.com.* Accessed August, 2017.

Chapter 4

1. McKeown, N., et al. Whole and refined-grain intakes are differentially associated with abdominal visceral and subcutaneous adiposity in healthy results: the Framingham Heart Study. *American Journal of Clinical Nutrition*, November 2010.
2. Preidt, R. Could white bread be making you fat? *WebMD*, May 2014.
3. Beddoe, A. *Biologic Ionization as Applied to Human Nutrition.* Wendell Whitman Co. 2012.
4. Schwalfenberg, G. The alkaline diet: Is there evidence that an alkaline pH diet benefits health? *Journal of Environmental and Public Health*, October 2012.
5. Enig, M. Mono and di-glycerides. *Weston A. Price Foundation, Wise Traditions in Food, farming and the Healing Arts.* Fall 2004.
6. Sanchez, M., and Parrott, W. Characterization of scientific studies usually cited as evidence of adverse effects of GM food/feed. *Plant Biotechnology Journal.* October 2017.
7. Thompson, L., et al. Phytoestrogen content of foods consumed in Canada, including isoflavones, lignans, and coumestan. *Nutrition and Cancer*, February 2006.
8. _____. What you need to know about GMO. Kaiser Permanente, *Partners in Health*, Fall 2012.

9. Formby, B., et al. Progesterone inhibits growth and induces apoptosis in breast cancer cells: inverse effects of Bel-2 and p53. *National Center for Biotechnology Information*, November-December 1998.
10. Weil, A. Dr. Weil's anti-inflammatory food pyramid – fact sheet. *Dr. Weil.com.*, accessed March 2017.
11. Bosetti. C., et al. A pooled analysis of case-control studies of thyroid cancer. VII. Cruciferous and other vegetables. *Cancer Center Control*, October 2002.
12. Dal Maso, L., et al. Risk factors for thyroid cancer: An epidemiological review focused on nutritional factors. *Cancer Center Control*, February 2009.
13. Derouiche, A., et al. Effect of argan and olive oil consumption on the hormonal profile of androgens among healthy adult Moroccan men. *National Product Communications*, January 2013.
14. Flynn, M., and Reinert, S. Comparing an olive oil-enriched diet to a standard lower-fat diet for weight loss in breast cancer survivors: a pilot study. *Journal of Women's Health*, June 2010.
15. Chang, C., et al. Essential fatty acids and human brain. *Acta Neurologica Taiwanica*, December 2009.
16. Owens-Liston, P. Study links sugar-sweetened soda to higher estrogen levels. *Health University of Utah, Health Feed*, March 2013.

Chapter 5

1. Arsenescu, V., et al. Polychlorinated biphenyl-77 induces adipocyte differentiation and pro-inflammatory adipokines and promotes obesity and atherosclerosis. *Environmental Health Perspectives*, June 2008.
2. Lim, J., et al. Inverse associations between long-term weight change and serum concentrations of persistent organic pollutants. *International Journal of Obesity*, September 2008.
3. Morales, E., et al. Influence of glutathione S-Transference polymorphisms on cognitive functioning effects induced by pp-DDT among preschoolers. *Environmental Health Perspectives*, November 2008.

4. Agatston, A., *The South Beach Diet: The Delicious, Doctor-Designed, Foolproof Plan for Fast and Healthy Weight Loss*. St. Martin's Paperbacks. 2003.

5. Yang, Q. Gain weight by "going diet?" Artificial sweeteners and the neurobiology of sugar cravings. *Yale Journal of Biology and Medicine*, June 2010.

6. Wilks, D., et al. Objectively measured physical activity and fat mass in children: A bias: adjusted meta-analysis of prospective studies. *PLOS one*, February 2011.

7. Jones, D., et al. Diet or exercise interventions vs combined behavioral weight management programs: A systematic review and meta-analysis of direct comparisons. *Journal of the Academy of Nutrition and Dietetics*, October 2014.

8. Pontzer, H., et al. Constrained total energy expenditure and metabolic adaption to physical activity in adult humans. *Current Biology*, January 2016.

9. Prado, A., and Airoldi, C. Toxic effect caused on microflora of soil by pesticide picloram applications. *Journal of Environmental Monitoring*, August 2001.

10. Dethefsen, L., and Relman, D. Incomplete recovery and individualized responses of the human distal gut microbiota to repeated antibiotic perturbation. *Proceedings of the National Academy of Sciences*, March 2011.

11. Vijay-Kumar, M., et al. Metabolic syndrome and altered gut microbiotica in mice lacking toll-like receptor 5. *Science*, April 2010.

12. Wallis, C. How gut bacteria help make us fat and thin. *Scientific American*, June 2014.

13. _____. Are antibiotics making us fat? *University of California Berkeley Wellness*, February 2016.

14. Besten, G., The role of short-chain fatty acids in the interplay between diet, gut microbiota, and host energy metabolism. *Journal of Lipid Research*, January 2013.

15. Sommer, M., et al. Functional characterization of the antibiotic resistance reservoir in the human microflora. *Science*, August 2009.

16. Lunder, S., and Sharp, R. US seafood advise flawed on mercury, omega-3s. *Environmental Working Group Report*, January 2014.
17. Rocha, J., et al. Mercury toxicity. *Journal of Biomedicine and Biotechnology,* September 2012.
18. _____. Overview of food ingredients, additives, & colors. *FDA.gov/Food/Ingredients Packaging Labeling/Food Additives,* accessed February 2017.
19. Dennis, B. FDA finalizes voluntary rules on phasing out certain antibiotics in livestock. *The Washington Post,* December 2013.
20. Cogliani, C., et al. Restricting antimicrobial use in food animals: Lessons from Europe. *Tufts University Microbe Magazine,* January 2011.
21. Ibid. *University of California Berkeley Wellness.*
22. Jeong, S., et al. Risk assessment of growth hormones and antimicrobial residues in meat. *Toxicological Research,* December 2010.
23. Saari, A. et al. Antibiotic exposure in infancy and risk of being overweight in first 24 months of life. *AAP Gateway,* April 2015.
24. Harth, R. Fish tale: new study evaluates antibiotic content in farm-raised fish. *Arizona State University Biodesign Institute,* October 2014.
25. Daley, C., et al. A review of fatty acid profiles and antioxidant content in grass-fed and grain-fed beef, *Nutrition Journal,* March 2010.
26. Lazic, M., et al. Reduced dietary omega-6 to omega-3 fatty acid ratio and 12/15-Lipoxygenase deficiency are protective against chronic high fat diet-induced steatohepatitis. *PLOS one,* September 2014.
27. _____. Potentially toxic chemicals detected in irradiated ground beef; Consumer groups urge FDA ban. *Public Citizen,* November 2003.
28. Schlosser, E. Cheap food nation. *Sierra Club Environmental Update,* November-December 2006.
29. _____. USDA FSIS Directive. Safe and suitable ingredients used in the production of meat, poultry, and egg products. *FSIS.USDA.gov.,* April 2013.

30. Bouvard, V., et al. Carcinogenicity of consumption of red and processed meat. *The Lancet Oncology*, December 2015.
31. Philpott, T. A brief history of our deadly addiction to nitrogen fertilizer. *Mother Jones*, April 2013.
32. _____. Whole grain resources for the national school lunch and school breakfast programs. *FNS.USDA.gov.*, accessed January 2018.
33. _____. Arsenic-based animal drugs and poultry. *FDA.gov.*, accessed April 2017.
34. Djousse, L., and Gaziano, J. Dietary cholesterol and coronary artery disease: A systematic review. *Current Atherosclerosis Reports*, November 2009.
35. _____. ERF: The making of a public health crisis. *Environmental Research Foundation*, August 1994.
36. Epstein, S. *What's In Your Milk?* Trafford Press, 2007.
37. Storrs, C. Hormones in food: *Huffington Post*, May 2011.
38. Hursting, S, et al. Obesity, energy balance and cancer: New opportunities for prevention. *National Center for Biotechnology Information*, November 2012.
39. _____. *United States Department of Agriculture. Tomatoes: Pesticide Data Program*, January 2016.
40. Kandyala, R., et al. Xylene: An overview of its health hazards and preventative measures. *Journal of Oral and Maxillofacial Pathology*, January-June 2010.
41. _____. N-Amyl acetate, human health effects, *Toxnet.nim.nih.gov*, accessed April 2018.
42. Bocarsly, M., et al. High-fructose corn syrup causes characteristics of obesity in rats: Increased body weight, body fat and triglyceride levels. *Pharmacology, Biochemistry and Behavior*, November 2010.
43. Neltner, T., et al. Data gaps in toxicity testing of chemicals allowed in food in the United States. *Reproductive Toxicology*, December 2013.
44. Jacobson, M. First-ever study reveals amounts of food dyes in brand-name foods. *Center for Science in the Public Interest*, May 2014.

Chapter 6

1. Frye, C., et al. Endocrine disruptors: A review of some sources, effects, and mechanisms of actions on behavior and neuroendocrine systems. *Journal of Neuro-Endocrinology,* January 2012.
2. Lim, S., et al. Chronic exposure to the herbicide atrazine causes mitochondrial dysfunction and insulin resistance. *PLOS one,* April 2009.
3. Lohr, A., and Gingerly, J. Chemical exposure linked to rising diabetes and obesity risk. *International Endocrine Society,* September 2015.
4. Diamanti-Kandarakis, E., et al. Endocrine-disrupting chemicals: An endocrine society scientific statement. *Endocrine Reviews,* June 2009.
5. Lah, K. Effects of pesticides on human health. *Toxipedia.org.,* May 2011.
6. Heindel, J. Endocrine disruptors and the obesity epidemic. *Oxford Journals/Toxicological Sciences,* October 2003.
7. _____. Dirty dozen endocrine disruptors: 12 hormone altering chemicals and how to avoid them. *Environmental Working Group.org.,* October 2013.
8. _____. TEDX list of potential endocrine disruptors. *Endocrine Disruption Exchange,* June 2015.
9. Minf, W. Effect of endocrine disruptor pesticides: A review. *National Center for Biotechnology Information,* June 2011.
10. Ravnskov, U. The cholesterol myths: Exposing the fallacy that saturated fat and cholesterol cause heart disease. *Newstrends Publishing,* 2000.
11. Bar-El Dadon, S., and Reifen, R. Soy as an endocrine Disruptor: Cause for Caution? *Journal of Pediatric Endocrinology & Metabolism,* September 2010.
12. Newbold, R., et al. Environmental estrogens and obesity. *Molecular and Cellular Endocrinology,* March 2009.
13. Vandenberg, L., et al. Hormones and endocrine disrupting chemicals: Low-dose effects and nonmonotonic dose responses. *Endocrine Reviews,* March 2012.

14. Cassidy, E. Extreme levels of herbicide Roundup found in food. *Environmental Working Group Review*, April 2014.

15. Samsel, A., and Seneff, S. Glyphosate's suppression of cytochrome P450 enzymes and amino acid biosynthesis by the gut microbiome: Pathways to modern diseases. *Entropy*, April 2013.

16. Teitelbaum, S., et al. Associations between phthalate metabolite urinary concentrations and body size measurements in New York City children. *Science Digest*, January 2012.

17. Oktar, S., et al. The relationship between phthalates and obesity; serum and urinary concentrations of phthalates. *National Center for Biotechnology Information*, January 2014.

18. Ibid, Lim.

19. Rattner, R. Pesticide turns male frog into females. *Live Science*, March 2010.

20. Wu, T., et al. Still poisoning the well: Atrazine continues to contaminate surface water and drinking water in the United States. *NRDC.org.*, April 2010.

21. Eskenazi, B., et al. Exposures of children to organophosphate pesticides and their potential adverse health effects. *Environmental Health Perspectives*, June 1999.

22. Lal, B., et al. Malathion exposure induces the endocrine disruption and growth retardation in the catfish, Clarias batrachus. *General and Comparative Endocrinology*, November 2012.

23. Yang, M., et al. Endocrine disrupting chemicals: human exposure and health risks. *Journal of Environmental Science and Health,* February 2006.

24. Mitchell, J., et al. Effect of a phytoestrogen food supplement on reproductive health in normal males. *Clinical Science*, May 2001

25. Donato, F., and Zani, C. Chronic exposure of organochlorine compounds and health effects in adults: diabetes and thyroid diseases. *National Center for Biotechnology Information*, May 2010.

26. Tuyet-Hanh, T., et al. Environmental health risk assessment of dioxin exposure. *National Center for Biotechnology Information,* May-June 2010.

27. Lau, C., et al. Perfluoroalkyl acids: A review of monitoring and toxicological findings. *Toxicological Sciences*, May 2007.
28. _____. Perflurochemicals (PFCs). America's Children and the Environment, Third Edition. *EPA.gov.*, accessed March 2017.

Chapter 7

1. Cuddy, A., et al. The benefit of power posing before a high-stakes social evaluation. *Harvard Business School Working Paper*, No. 13-027, September 2012.
2. Daubenmier, J., et al. Mindfulness intervention for stress eating and to reduce cortisol and abdominal fat among overweight and obese women: An exploratory randomized controlled study. *Journal of Obesity*, October 2011.
3. Chevalier, G., et al. Earthing: health implications of reconnecting the human body to the earth's surface electrons. *Alternative and Complementary Medicine,* January 2000.
4. Sokal, K., and Sokal, P. "Earthing the human body influences physiologic processes. *Journal of Alternative and Complementary Medicine*, April 2011.
5. Ghaly, M., and Teplitz, D. The biologic effects of grounding the human body during sleep as measured by cortisol levels and subjective reporting of sleep, pain, and stress. Journal of *Alternative and Complementary Medicine*, October 2004.
6. Lesinski, M., et al. Dose-Response Relationships of Balance Training in Healthy Young Adults: A systematic Review and Meta-Analysis, *Sports Medicine*, April 2015.
7. Ross, A., et al, A Different Weight Loss Experience: A Qualitative Study Exploring the Behavior, Physical, and Psychosocial Changes Associated with Yoga That Promote Weight Loss. *Evidence-Based Complementary and Alternative Medicine*, August 2015.
8. Gandevia, S. and Proske, U., Proprioception: The Sense Within. *The Scientist*, September 2016.
9. Dickinson, J. *Proprioceptive Control of Human Movement*. Princeton Book Co. 1976.

10. Victor, M. and Roper A., et al. *Adams and Victor's Principles of Neurology, Chapter 9. Seventh Edition.* McGraw-Hill Professional: 2000.
11. Rogge, AK, et al. Balance training improves memory and spatial cognition in healthy adults. *Scientific Reports*, July 2017.

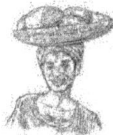

BIBLIOGRAPHY

_____. Abdominal fat and what to do about it. Harvard Medical School, *Harvard Health Publications*, October 2015.

_____. Are antibiotics making us fat? University of California Berkeley *Wellness*, February 2016.

_____. Arsenic-based animal drugs and poultry. *FDA.gov.*, accessed April 2017.

_____. Dirty dozen endocrine disruptors: 12 hormone altering chemicals and how to avoid them. *Environmental Working Group.org.*, October 2013.

_____. ERF: The making of a public health crisis. *Environmental Research Foundation*, August 1994.

_____. Global weight loss and gain market (2009 – 2014). *Marketsandmarkets.com.*, accessed February 2018.

_____. N-Amyl acetate, human health effects, *Toxnet.nim.nih.gov*, accessed April 2018.

_____.Obesity and overweight fast starts. *Centers for Disease Control and Prevention, cdc.gov/nchs.*, accessed February 2018.

_____. Overview of food ingredients, additives, & colors. *FDA.gov/Food/Ingredients Packaging Labeling/Food Additives*, accessed February 2017.

_____. Perflurochemicals (PFCs). America's Children and the Environment, Third Edition. *EPA.gov.*, accessed March 2017.

_____. Potentially toxic chemicals detected in irradiated ground beef; Consumer groups urge FDA ban. *Public Citizen*, November 2003.

_____. TEDX list of potential endocrine disruptors. *Endocrine Disruption Exchange*, June 2015.

_____. United States Department of Agriculture. *Tomatoes: Pesticide Data Program*, January 2016.

_____. USDA FSIS Directive. Safe and suitable ingredients used in the production of meat, poultry, and egg products. *FSIS.USDA.gov.*, April 2013.

_____. What you need to know about GMO. Kaiser Permanente, *Partners in Health*, Fall 2012.

_____.Whole grain resources for the national school lunch and school breakfast programs. *FNS.USDA.gov.*, accessed January 2018.

Agatston, A., *The South Beach Diet: The Delicious, Doctor-Designed, Foolproof Plan for Fast and Healthy Weight Loss*. St. Martin's Paperbacks. 2003.

Arsenescu, V., et al. Polychlorinated biphenyl-77 induces adipocyte differentiation and pro- inflammatory adipokines and promotes obesity and atherosclerosis. *Environmental Health Perspectives*, June 2008.

Bar-El Dadon, S., and Reifen, R. Soy as an endocrine Disruptor: Cause for Caution? *Journal of Pediatric Endocrinology and Metabolism*, September 2010.

Beddoe, A. *Biologic Ionization as Applied to Human Nutrition*. Wendell Whitman Co. 2012.

Besten, G., The role of short-chain fatty acids in the interplay between diet, gut microbiota, and host energy metabolism. *Journal of Lipid Research*, January 2013.

Bienerstock, J., et al. Ingestion of Lactobacillus strain regulates emotional behavior and central GABA receptor expression in a mouse via the vagus nerve. *Proceedings of the National Academy of Sciences*, July 2011.

Blanchette, K. *Prevention of the Disease of Aging*. Xulon Press, 2007.

Blumberg, B., and Loberg, K. *The Obesogen Effect: Why We Eat Less and Exercise More but Still Struggle to Lose Weight*. Grand Central Life & Style, 2018.

Bocarsly, M., et al. High-fructose corn syrup causes characteristics of obesity in rats: Increased body weight, body fat and triglyceride levels. *Pharmacology, Biochemistry and Behavior*, November 2010.

Bosetti. C., et al. A pooled analysis of case-control studies of thyroid cancer. VII. Cruciferous and other vegetables. *Cancer Causes Control*, October 2002.

Bouvard, V., et al. Carcinogenicity of consumption of red and processed meat. *The Lancet Oncology*, December 2015.

Cassidy, E. Extreme levels of herbicide Roundup found in food. *Environmental Working Group Review*, April 2014.

Chevalier, G., et al. Earthing: health implications of reconnecting the human body to the earth's surface electrons. *Alternative and Complementary Medicine,* January 2000.

Cogliani, C., et al. Restricting antimicrobial use in food animals: Lessons from Europe. Tufts University *Microbe Magazine*, January 2011.

Cuddy, A., et al. The benefit of power posing before a high-stakes social evaluation. *Harvard Business School Working Paper No. 13-027*, September 2012.

Dal Maso, L., et al. Risk factors for thyroid cancer: An epidemiological review focused on nutritional factors. *Cancer Center Control*, February 2009.

Daley, C., et al. A review of fatty acid profiles and antioxidant content in grass-fed and grain-fed beef, *Nutrition Journal*, March 2010.

Daubenmier, J., et al. Mindfulness intervention for stress eating and to reduce cortisol and abdominal fat among overweight and obese women: An exploratory randomized controlled study. *Journal of Obesity*, October 2011.

Dennis, B. FDA finalizes voluntary rules on phasing out certain antibiotics in livestock. *The Washington Post*, December 11, 2013.

Derouiche, A., et al. Effect of argan and olive oil consumption on the hormonal profile of androgens among healthy adult Moroccan men. *National Center for Biotechnology Information*, January 2013.

Dethefsen, L., and Relman, D. Incomplete recovery and individualized responses of the human distal gut microbiota to repeated antibiotic perturbation. *Proceedings of the National Academy of Sciences*, March 2011.

Diamanti-Kandarakis, E., et al. Endocrine-disrupting chemicals: An endocrine society scientific statement. *Endocrine Reviews*, June 2009.

Dickinson, J. *Proprioceptive Control of Human Movement*. Princeton Book Co. 1976.

Djousse, L., and Gaziano, J. Dietary cholesterol and coronary artery disease: A systematic review. *Current Atherosclerosis Reports*, November 2009.

Donato, F., and Zani, C. Chronic exposure of organochlorine compounds and health effects in adults: diabetes and thyroid diseases. *National Center for Biotechnology Information*, May 2010.

Enig, M. Mono and di-glycerides. Weston A. Price Foundation, *Wise Traditions in Food, farming and the Healing Arts*, Fall 2004.

Epstein, S. *What's In Your Milk?* Trafford Press, 2007.

Eskenazi, B., et al. Exposures of children to organophosphate pesticides and their potential adverse health effects. *Environmental Health Perspectives*, June 1999.

Formby, B., et al. Progesterone inhibits growth and induces apoptosis in breast cancer cells: inverse effects of Bel-2 and p53. *National Center for Biotechnology Information*, November-December 1998.

Frye, C., et al. Endocrine disruptors: A review of some sources, effects, and mechanisms of actions on behavior and neuroendocrine systems. *Journal of Neuro-Endocrinology*, January 2012.

Fung, J. The role of fibre I-hormone obesity. *Intensive Dietary Management*, May 2014.

Gandevia, S. and Proske, U., Proprioception: The sense within. *The Scientist*, September 2016.

Ghaly, M., and Teplitz, D. The biologic effects of grounding the human body during sleep as measured by cortisol levels and subjective reporting of sleep, pain, and stress. *Journal of Alternative and Complementary Medicine*, October 2004.

Gottfried, S. 10 Surprising facts about how hormones disrupt your health and weight. *Dr. Sara Gottfried.com.*, accessed December 2017.

Grun, F., and Blumberg, B. Minireview: The case for obesogens. *Molecular Endocrinology*, August 2009.

Harth, R. Fish tale: new study evaluates antibiotic content in farm-raised fish. *Arizona State University Biodesign Institute*, October 2014.

Harvie, M., et al. The effects of intermittent or continuous energy restriction on weight loss and metabolic risk disease markers: A randomized trial in young overweight women. *International Journal of Obesity*, May 2010.

Heindel, J. Endocrine disruptors and the obesity epidemic. *Oxford Journals/Toxicological Sciences*, October 2003.

Hursting, S, et al. Obesity, energy balance and cancer: New opportunities for prevention. *National Center for Biotechnology Information*, November 2012.

Jacobson, M. First-ever study reveals amounts of food dyes in brand-name foods. *Center for Science in the Public Interest*, May 2014.

Jeong, S., et al. Risk assessment of growth hormones and antimicrobial residues in meat. *Toxicological Research*, December 2010.

Jin Noh, H., et al. The relationship between hippocampal volume and cognition in patients with chronic primary insomnia. *Journal of Clinical Neurology*, June 2012.

Jones, D., et al. Diet or exercise interventions vs combined behavioral weight management programs: A systematic review and meta-analysis of direct comparisons. *Journal of the Academy of Nutrition and Dietetics*, October 2014.

Kandyala, R., et al. Xylene: An overview of its health hazards and preventative measures. *Journal of Oral and Maxillofacial Pathology*, January-June 2010.

Lah, K. Effects of pesticides on human health. *Toxipedia.org.*, May 2011.

Lal, B., et al. Malathion exposure induces the endocrine disruption and growth retardation in the catfish, Clarias batrachus. *General and Comparative Endocrinology*, November 2012.

Lally, P., et al. How are habits formed: Modeling habit formation in the real world. *European Journal of Social Psychology*, July 2009.

Lally, P., et al. Making health habitual: The psychology of 'habit-formation' and general practice. *The British Journal of General Practice*, December 2012.

Lau, C., et al. Perfluoroalkyl acids: A review of monitoring and toxicological findings. *Toxicological Sciences*, May 2007.

Lazic, M., et al. Reduced dietary omega-6 to omega-3 fatty acid ratio and 12/15-Lipoxygenase deficiency are protective against chronic high fat diet-induced steatohepatitis. *PLOS one*, September 2014.

Lesinski, M., et al. Dose-response relationships of balance training in healthy young adults: A systematic review and meta-analysis. *Sports Medicine*, April 2015.

Lim, J., et al. Inverse associations between long-term weight change and serum concentrations of persistent organic pollutants. *International Journal of Obesity*, September 2008.

Lim, S., et al. Chronic exposure to the herbicide atrazine causes mitochondrial dysfunction and insulin resistance. *PLOS one*, April 2009.

Lohr, A., and Gingerly, J. Chemical exposure linked to rising diabetes and obesity risk. *International Endocrine Society*, September 2015.

Lunder, S., and Sharp, R. US seafood advise flawed on mercury, omega- 3s. *Environmental Working Group Report*, January 2014.

MacKelvie, K., et al. Bone mineral density and serum testosterone in chronically trained, high mileage 40-55 year old male runners. *British Journal of Sports Medicine*, August 2000.

Mann, T., et al. Medicare's search for effective obesity treatments: diets are not the answer. *American Psychologist*, April 2007.

Marquart, M. Defective joy gene: Study finds Germans incapable of enjoying life. *Spiegel Online International*, May 2012.

McKeown, N., et al. Whole and refined-grain intakes are differentially associated with abdominal visceral and subcutaneous adiposity in healthy results: the Framingham Heart Study. *American Journal of Clinical Nutrition*, November 2010.

Minf, W. Effect of endocrine disruptor pesticides: A review. *National Center for Biotechnology Information*, June 2011.

Mitchell, J., et al. Effect of a phytoestrogen food supplement on reproductive health in normal males. *Clinical Science*, May 2001.

Morales, E., et al. Influence of glutathione S-Transference polymorphisms on cognitive functioning effects induced by pp-DDT among preschoolers. *Environmental Health Perspectives*, November 2008.

Morgentaler, A. Harvard expert shares his thoughts on testosterone-replacement therapy. Harvard Medical School, *Harvard Health Publications*, February 2011.

Mozaffarian, D., et al. Changes in diet and lifestyle and long-term weight gain in women and men. *New England Journal of Medicine*, June 2011.

Neltner, T., et al. Data gaps in toxicity testing of chemicals allowed in food in the United States. *Reproductive Toxicology*, December 2013.

Newbold, R., et al. Environmental estrogens and obesity. *Molecular and Cellular Endocrinology*, March 2009.

Oktar, S., et al. The relationship between phthalates and obesity; serum and urinary concentrations of phthalates. *National Center for Biotechnology Information*, January 2014.

Owens-Liston, P. Study links sugar-sweetened soda to higher estrogen levels. Health University of Utah, *Health Feed*, March 2013.

Peeke, P., *Body for Life for Women: A Woman's Plan for Physical and Mental Transformation*. Rodale Books, 2009.

Philpott, T. A brief history of our deadly addiction to nitrogen fertilizer. *Mother Jones*, April 2013.

Pietilainen, K., et al. Does dieting make you fat? A twin study. *International Journal of Obesity*, March 2012.

Pontzer, H., et al. Constrained total energy expenditure and metabolic adaption to physical activity in adult humans. *Current Biology*, January 2016.

Prado, A., and Airoldi, C. Toxic effect caused on microflora of soil by pesticide picloram applications. *Journal of Environmental Monitoring*, August 2001.

Preidt, R. Could white bread be making you fat? *WebMD*, May 2014.

Prior, A., et al. Cholesterol, coconuts and diet on Polynesian atolls: a natural experiment. *American Journal of Clinical Nutrition*, 1981.

Rattner, R. Pesticide turns male frog into females. *Live Science*, March 2010.

Ravnskov, U. *The cholesterol myths: Exposing the fallacy that saturated fat and cholesterol cause heart disease*. Newstrends Publishing, 2000.

Rind, R. Addressing thyroid and adrenal insufficiency. *Weston A. Price Foundation*, June 2009.

Rocha, J., et al. Mercury toxicity. *Journal of Biomedicine and Biotechnology*, September 2012.

Rogge, AK, et al. Balance training improves memory and spatial cognition in healthy adults. *Scientific Reports*, July 2017.

Ross, A., et al, A Different weight loss experience: A qualitative study exploring the behavior, physical, and psychosocial changes associated with yoga that promote weight loss. *Evidence-Based Complementary and Alternative Medicine*, August 2015.

Russell, WR, et al. High-protein, reduced-carbohydrate weight-loss diets promote metabolite profiles likely to be detrimental to colonic health. *American Journal of Clinical Nutrition*, May 2011.

Saad, F., et al. Testosterone as potential effective therapy in treatment of obesity in men with testosterone deficiency: A review. *Current Diabetes Reviews*, March 2012.

Saari, A. et al. Antibiotic exposure in infancy and risk of being overweight in first 24 months of life. *AAP Gateway*, April 2015.

Sahelian, R. Oxytocin hormone natural ways to increase; benefits and side effects. *Dr. Ray Sahelian.com.*, accessed June 2017.

Samsel, A., and Seneff, S. Glyphosate's suppression of cytochrome P450 enzymes and amino acid biosynthesis by the gut microbiome: Pathways to modern diseases. *Entropy*, April 2013.

Sanchez, M., and Parrott, W. Characterization of scientific studies usually cited as evidence of adverse effects of GM food/feed. *Plant Biotechnology Journal*, October 2017.

Sartorelli, D., et al. High intake of fruits and vegetables predicts weight loss in Brazilian overweight adults. *Nutrition Research Journal*, April 2008.

Sawyer, BJ., et al. Predictors of fat mass changes in response to aerobic exercise training in women. *Journal of Strength and Conditioning Research*, February 2015.

Schlosser, E. Cheap food nation. *Sierra Club Environmental Update*, November-December 2006.

Schwalfenberg, G. The alkaline diet: Is there evidence that an alkaline pH diet benefits health? *Journal of Environmental and Public Health*, October 2012.

Secor, E., et al. Bromelain inhibits allergic sensitization and murine asthma via modulation of dendritic cells. *Evidence Based Complementary Alternative Medicine*, December 2013.

Sokal, K., and Sokal, P. Earthing the human body influences physiologic processes, *Journal of Alternative and Complementary Medicine*, April 2011.

Sommer, M., et al. Functional characterization of the antibiotic resistance reservoir in the human microflora. *Science*, August 2009.

Stenblom, EL., et al. Consumption of thylakoid-rich spinach extract reduces hunger, increases satiety and reduces cravings for palatable food in overweight women. *Elsevier*, August 2015.

Storrs, C. Hormones in food: Should you worry? *Huffington Post*, May 2011.

Streeter, C., et al. Effects of yoga versus walking on mood, anxiety, and brain GABA levels: A randomized controlled MRS study. Journal of *Alternative and Complementary Medicine*, November 2010.

Surninski, R., et al. Acute effect of amino acid ingestion and resistance exercise on plasma growth hormone concentration in young me. *International Journal of Sport Nutrition*, July 1997.

Teitelbaum, S., et al. Associations between phthalate metabolite urinary concentrations and body size measurements in New York City children. *Science Digest*, January 2012.

Thompson, L., et al. Phytoestrogen content of foods consumed in Canada, including isoflavones, lignans, and coumestan. *Nutrition and Cancer*, February 2006.

Tuyet-Hanh, T., et al. Environmental health risk assessment of dioxin exposure. *National Center for Biotechnology Information*, May-June 2010.

Vandenberg, L., et al. Hormones and endocrine disrupting chemicals: Low-dose effects and nonmonotonic dose responses. *Endocrine Reviews*, March 2012.

Victor M. and Roper A., et al. *Adams and Victor's Principles of Neurology, Chapter 9. Seventh Edition*. McGraw-Hill Professional: 2000.

Vijay-Kumar, M., et al. Metabolic syndrome and altered gut microbiotica in mice lacking toll-like receptor 5. *Science*, April 2010.

Wallis, C. How gut bacteria help make us fat and thin. *Scientific American*, June 2014.

Wang, C., and Liao, JK. A mouse model of diet-induced obesity and insulin resistance. Methods in Molecular Biology, *Springer Science Media*, 2012.

Wang, C., et al. Low-fat high-fiber diet decreased serum and urine androgens in men. *Journal of Clinical Endocrinology and Metabolism*, June 2005.

Wang, S., et al. Resveratrol induces brown-like adipocyte formation in white fat through activation of AMP-activated protein kinase (AMPK) a1. *International Journal of Obesity*, October 2015.

Weil, A. Dr. Weil's anti-inflammatory food pyramid – fact sheet. *Dr. Weil.com.*, accessed March 2017.

Westererp-Plantenga, M., et al. Metabolic effects of spices, teas, and caffeine. *Physiology and Behavior*, August 2006.

Wilks, D., et al. Objectively measured physical activity and fat mass in children: A bias: adjusted meta-analysis of prospective studies. *PLOS one*, February 2011.

Wilson, J. *Adrenal Fatigue: The 21st Century Stress Syndrome*. Smart Publications 2001.

Wilson, J., et al. Concurrent training: A meta-analysis examining interference of aerobic and existence exercise. *Journal of Strength and Conditioning Research*, August 2012.

Wu, A., et al. Tea and circulating estrogen levels in postmenopausal Chinese women in Singapore. *Oxford Journals, Molecular Carcinogenesis*, May 2005.

Wu., K., et al. Still poisoning the well: Atrazine continues to contaminate surface water and drinking water in the United States. *NRDC.org.*, April 2010.

Yang, M., et al. Endocrine disrupting chemicals: human exposure and health risks. *Journal of Environmental Science and Health*, February 2006.

Yang, Q. Gain weight by "going diet?" Artificial sweeteners and the neurobiology of sugar cravings. *Yale Journal of Biology and Medicine*, June 2010.

Young, E. The dark side of oxytocin, much more than just a "love hormone." *Discover Science*, November 2010.

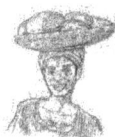

INDEX

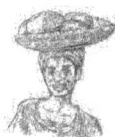

Index of Relevant Websites

Drberg.com
Drhyman.com
Drpeeke.com
Ewg.org
Garytaubes.com
Marksdailyapple.com
Michaelpollan.com
Robertlustig.com
Saragottfriedmd.com
Westonpriceaprice.org
Wheatbelly.com
Drweil.com
Drmercola.com

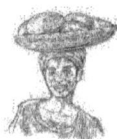

About the author

Randy Smythe is a legendary sports training expert. His expertise in developing speed in elite sports has put him at the forefront of athletic training on the field and in lecture rooms. He has coached for the Dallas Cowboys, Chicago Bears, Milwaukee Brewers, many international professional soccer teams, and Grand Slam tennis champions. His writing about elite training and nutrition has been published in numerous sports journals and brought him to 23 foreign nations as a speaker and consultant.

In 2007 with *Baseball Speed Training*, Randy Smythe created the bible of speed development in the sport. His 2009 book, *Feeding Your Wild Child*, put him in the forefront of nutrition controversy as he proposed a complete natural food treatment program for ADHD children. His 2012 book for elite athletic development, *The Speed Power Diet*, similarly proved controversial as he proposed highly specialized nutrition as a way to compete against athletes who use performance enhancing drugs.

Over decades of work and teaching, he has worked with generations of adults seeking his unique methods of health and weightloss.

Randy lives and works in South Florida. He was educated at the University of California, Berkeley, and went on to get his master's degree in sport training and nutrition. Many of his myth-shattering concepts for adult nutrition and weightloss come from decades of trial and error work with world class athletes.

Feel free to contact him at www.carefreecaribbean.com.

www.ingramcontent.com/pod-product-compliance
Lightning Source LLC
Chambersburg PA
CBHW031155270326
41931CB00006B/275